COVID-19: LIFE-SAVING STRATEGIES THE NEWS MEDIA WILL NEVER TELL YOU

Paul Thomas, M.D.
www.DrPaulApproved.com

Published Internationally by Dr. Paul Approved
Portland, Oregon

© 2020 Paul Thomas, M.D.

ISBN 978-1-71693-797-2

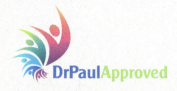

Dedicated to my friend Bud and all who are suffering from the COVID-19 coronavirus

---

"The only thing to fear is fear itself"
  -FDR

"May your choices reflect your hopes, not your fears."
  -Nelson Mandela

My hope is that this book will empower you.

Knowledge is power.

The unknown and the ridiculous messaging, coming from most sources, is that all you can do is shut yourself in your house and wait a year or more for a vaccine to come and save you. This is stoking anxiety and fear.

This book will empower you with the exact information you need and concrete tools to survive COVID-19 should you happen to get it and become really ill.

You will have the tools to be a warrior and go to battle with confidence and courage. Control your fear and be willing to take action. Don't just read this book. Use the information to get the tools you need to go into battle if that time comes.

Disclaimer:

All information in this E-book and otherwise shared by author Paul Thomas MD is for general guidance and informational purposes only. Readers are encouraged to confirm the information provided with other sources. Patients and consumers should review the information carefully with their professional health care provider. The information is not intended to replace medical advice offered by other physicians. Please check with your medical providers before trying anything that you may have learned here.

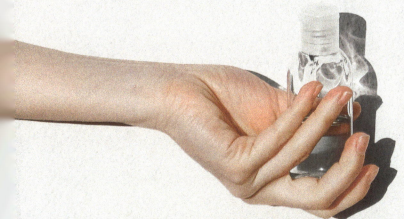

Paul Thomas MD, author, is writing this using the best information available at this moment. We are early in the pandemic and more shall be revealed. Take what makes sense, and leave the rest. Use what you can and when some of the information in this book becomes obsolete due to new information - disregard it!

Table of Contents

DrPaulApproved

Introduction

06	Opening Remarks
07	Introduction

Part A: What to do

09	The most important thing you can do to avoid getting infected
10	Emergency Respiratory & Immune Rescue Kit
12	Fear
14	Time to get healthy
15	Taking your health into your own hands
16	Avoid Covid-19 exposure & Boost your Immune System
22	How to know when it is time to go to the hospital
23	What to do when you have a COVID-19 infection
25	Please take Covid-19 seriously
28	Working together in Community
29	Respiratory rescue kit
29	Coronavirus treatment kit

Part B: The Science

31	The Virus
33	How the virus enters the body & replicates
34	Keeping COVID-19 out of your house
35	Symptoms
38	The China Experience
39	The USA
40	Flattening the curve

Treatment Options

42	Vitamin C
46	Melatonin
48	Vitamin D
51	Magnesium and Zinc
52	CBD
52	Selenium
53	Pharmaceuticals

Table of Contents

Stories

54   Bud

56   New Orleans ER Doctor Tells it Like it is

Summary- Putting things in Perspective

59   Thoughts

63   The Rush for a Vaccine

67   Final Thoughts

References

72   References

Appendix A

79   Appendix A

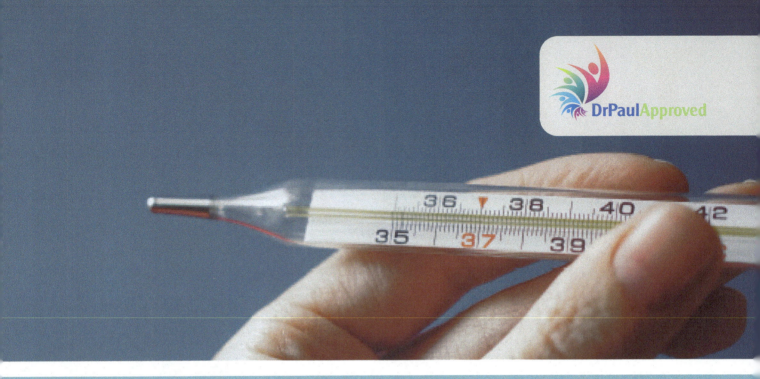

OPENING STATEMENT

Many if not most of us have friends and family who either may have the COVID-19 illness or have tested positive for SARS- CoV-2. Perhaps you have loved ones who are elderly or immunocompromised or with significant underlying health issues making them most vulnerable. My heart goes out to everyone around the globe suffering due to this disease. I'm inspired once again by the countless professionals and volunteers risking their lives to help those in need.

We need calm and humility. Stress is an under appreciated risk factor when it comes to harming our immune systems, and nothing could be worse than the panic so many are feeling. Remember that just as the virus is contagious, so are emotions. I've written this book quickly because it offers knowledge and specific "do this" information that can give you that sense of calm that you need to move through this crisis. I submit with humility that in just days, weeks or months, some of what is in this book will be obsolete as better information becomes available.

Note that this book is not intended to be a health claim for any dietary supplement. As of this writing, no pharmaceutical drug or any dietary supplement has been proven in long-term placebo controlled studies to treat COVID-19.

INTRODUCTION

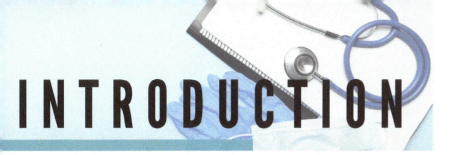
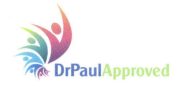

My friend Bud is hospitalized a few miles down the road from me. He is in quarantine, no-one, not even his wife can see him and all we can do is hear about his progressive slide toward death.

The Kawasaki Vulcan motorcycle I ride was Bud's. I was just with him a couple months ago at a meeting. Sadly, he went to the hospital before I knew he was even sick and was put in quarantine while awaiting the COVID-19 test results. They came back positive, and over the past week he has gone from being in a hospital room, to needing oxygen, to being placed in the ICU (Intensive Care Unit) where he has signed a DNR (Do Not Resuscitate) order and is likely going to need a ventilator any day now. The death rate for older men once on a ventilator appears to be very high, way over 50%.

What upsets me and is the reason I am rushing this E-book to the world, is that THERE ARE THINGS WE CAN DO to minimize the infection and help our immune system and body rid the infection. THESE THINGS MAY BE LIFESAVING, but they are not possible once you enter the world of mainstream medicine in the USA and probably in most countries. That's why it's crucial to read this book to discover what you can do to keep yourself and your loved ones healthy. These are strategies I use as a medical doctor with my patients as well as with my own family at home.

A BRIEF CLARIFICATION ON THE DIFFERENT NAMES BEING USED FOR THIS PANDEMIC

Coronavirus disease 2019 (COVID-19) is the name for the illness we are all hearing about. This virus is a coronavirus that has specifically been labeled SARS-CoV-2 which stands for severe acute respiratory syndrome coronavirus 2.

Take a look at the final thoughts at the end of this book for a perspective that is generally lacking in the media storm we are all being subjected to.

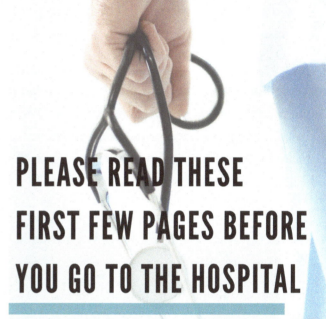

PLEASE READ THESE FIRST FEW PAGES BEFORE YOU GO TO THE HOSPITAL

On March 26, 2020, the U.S. surpassed China and Italy to become the nation with the most COVID-19 infections in the world. This despite the fact that we have only recently started testing and the outbreaks are just getting started in most areas. The Hopkins University dashboard showed the U.S. with 85,840 cases as of 11 p.m., ET, moving past Italy (80,589) and China (81,782), and more than 1,296 people have died in the U.S.

The information in this book is educational and Informational only: IT IS NOT MEDICAL ADVICE. It is not intended to diagnose or treat. No pharmaceutical or dietary supplement has been proven in long-term placebo-controlled studies to treat or prevent COVID-19.

PART A: WHAT TO DO

For hard science, you can read Part 2. However, I decided to jump right in with potentially useful suggestions in case you got lost in the science and gave up before getting to these tips, which could save your life. Nothing written in this book is meant to diagnose or treat and is just informational for you to review with your healthcare provider.

Please understand that this COVID-19 virus is new, unique and much more infectious and more fatal than anything we have experienced in generations. That said, a healthy immune system and a host of healthy lifestyle choices are the key to survival.

If you do what everyone else does you will get the results everyone else gets. We have clearly entered uncharted territory.

Day after day all the media outlets report bad to worse news: more infections, more deaths, shortages of vital supplies and changing recommendations from the CDC and public health officials, governors, the president, the surgeon general and world leaders. You would think there was nothing else happening in the world, other than coronavirus. A massive outbreak in China, then South Korea, then Italy and now throughout Europe exploded in the USA and arrived in your country and town. These same media outlets that have focused on politics to the exclusion of all else now have something even better: death, fear and a massive unknown to exploit.

The total blunder in testing has resulted in only the very ill getting tested which has propped up death rates which reach 1% - 3% and for those over 80 years old well over 10%. Please realize that in China a death rate of 4,000 out of 1.3 billion translates into a death rate of 1/350,000 people. Italy seems to be having the worst death rates although one report says that 99% of those dying had at least one underlying health condition. Numbers from Italy are so massive that they are now already at a death rate of over 1 person/1000 for their entire population. So, take this seriously!

On March 24 the local health system and hospital that I'm most engaged with sent out this information: "In the Oregon Region, test positivity rate is about 4.1% overall. Inpatient tests have a 5% positive rate; outpatients have 3.7% positive rate. To our knowledge, we have yet to see a caregiver or provider return with a positive test." This was at a time when testing has just been 600 a week and really only going on for the past week. The testing was limited to patients with symptoms, caregivers and providers. Clearly Oregon and the Portland area in particular is just at the beginning of this outbreak. The storm is ahead as is the case for much of the world.

For now, where I live you can say that at least 95% do not have COVID-19! But don't relax precautions – the tidal wave is likely coming to you anywhere in the world due to the contagiousness and rapid rate at which cases seem to double, once the virus is in a community. Doubling rates have been reported as high as every 2 to 3 days.

The information in this book is educational and Informational only: IT IS NOT MEDICAL ADVICE. It is not intended to diagnose or treat. No pharmaceutical or dietary supplement has been proven in long-term placebo-controlled studies to treat or prevent COVID-19.

The WHO Director-General Tedros Adhanom Ghebreyesus said on March 23, "The pandemic is accelerating" with more than 350,000 cases in the world. Tedros called for countries to cooperate: "We need to attack the virus with aggressive and targeted tactics." The article says that "it took 67 days to confirm the first hundred thousand cases, 11 days to confirm the second hundred thousand cases and just four days to confirm the third hundred thousand cases."

That said, if we ended up with 30,000 deaths in the USA, that would be a rate of 1/10,000. It will still be the most devastating pandemic of the past century. Some are predicting the number of USA deaths to be even worse than this.

Prepare, don't panic and do everything in your power to get as healthy as you possibly can. Do your best to reduce stress and the immune-harming effects of consuming sugar, processed foods and bad fats (and especially avoid partially hydrogenated vegetable oils).

I'm going to make a few recommendations in this book, of things you can do, supplements you should consider taking now and things to consider if infected and having symptoms. That said, please understand that the entire world is learning about this virus and what to do together. Ideas will change and new effective strategies will emerge. This book is not intended to be exhaustive and share every possible thought or remedy or approach. I am trying to bring to readers a quick response as that is what is required. Continue to research and learn. Nothing here is intended to diagnose or treat. The ideas presented here are what I am doing and what I recommend to my patients. They are something you may want to consider. These recommendations are informational. While taking them into consideration, pay attention to the latest research that will be exploding by the day.

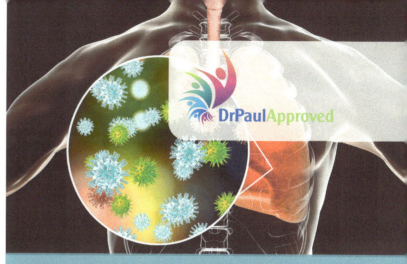

THE MOST IMPORTANT THING YOU CAN DO TO AVOID GETTING INFECTED:

First, before I present some approaches you won't hear about in the news media, I want to emphasize the importance of three basic yet effective strategies:

1. Keep your hands clean. Anytime you touch anything someone else might have touched assume you have COVID-19 on your hands. Wash every time.
2. Don't touch your face.

This infection is spread by fomites – the virus on surfaces that you touch and then self-inoculate to your face. Evidence suggests that very few cases, outside the hospital setting, are spread through the air. We know this because of the low rate of transmission within the homes of those quarantined in Wuhan, China. That said, wear a mask or cover your mouth and nose with a bandana when indoors with others who might have the infection, or you are in situations where social distancing is not possible.

3. Wear a mask when social distancing is not possible. Wear a mask or cover your mouth and nose with a bandana when indoors with others who might have the infection, and when you are in situations where social distancing is not possible. We know that this virus replicates in our throats.(1)

Given the large numbers of expiratory particles known to be emitted during breathing and speech, and how contagious COVID-19 is, it is possible that simple close contact conversations with an infected person, even if they he or she had no symptoms, could transmit COVID-19.(2)

The information in this book is educational and Informational only: IT IS NOT MEDICAL ADVICE. It is not intended to diagnose or treat. No pharmaceutical or dietary supplement has been proven in long-term placebo-controlled studies to treat or prevent COVID-19.

EMERGENCY RESPIRATORY AND IMMUNE RESCUE KIT

Symptoms of COVID-19 might include horrible fatigue, shortness of breath, severe nausea, coughing, fever or new unusual extreme problems that you haven't experience before. For anyone who is clearly developing lung problems or those severe symptoms from COVID-19 start implementing the following few measures as soon as you can.

EMERGENCY RESPIRATORY AND IMMUNE SUPPORT KIT

1. Nebulize Argentyn-23* 2 ml every 2 - 4 hours, breathing in as deep as you can (don't hyperventilate – very slow deep breaths)
2. Take 1,000 mg vitamin C every 30 minutes while awake (lower dose if severe diarrhea develops, and take it every 15 minutes if you are worse and close to needing a ventilator)
3. Take 0.5 to 1 mg melatonin every 4 hours during the day and 10 mg at bedtime
4. Take 50 – 200 mg CBD daily (divide into 2 - 4 doses a day)
5. Take SBI (Serum Bovine Immunoglobulin) up to 2.5 grams twice a day

If Argentyn 23* (23 ppm) is not available, Sovereign Silver is 10 ppm of the same fine particle silver solution that I have used extensively in clinical practice with my patients. If these are not available, consider other brands based on reputation and testing or the experience of other providers who use them.

While I have only mentioned using Argentyn 23 nebulized, since we know that SARS-CoV-2 replicates in the throat, particularly during the first 5 days of symptoms(3) it may be helpful to slow this infection by spraying Argentyn 23 on the back of the throat several times a day during the early phases when you just have a cold or scratchy throat. (Again, nothing in this book is intended to be a medical recommendation — just information and sharing of the science that we do have). SBI Protect is now marketed by OrthoMolecular (2.5 mg/dose). Enteragam (5mg/dose) is the equivalent and Megamucosa (1 mg/dose) has the same SBI ingredient along with a few others.

Most CBD products are made from hemp and marijuana plants and tend to be contaminated with some THC along with solvents used to extract the CBD and other toxins. There is a new CBD product made from oranges that is 99.5% pure. The remaining 0.5% is a terpene found in oranges. Terpenes are healthful components of certain plants. They are often responsible for the fragrance of the plants. This CBD product made from oranges is bioidentical to the CBD our bodies make and is the one I recommend. For access to my 25% wellevate professional discount on most products and more information on the new CBD product go to click.drpaulapproved.com

Read on for more specific instructions of things to do and not to do, to both prevent infection and to help your body's immune system so you can fight this thing if you get the virus. To discover the scientific basis for the suggestions I am making, you can jump to section 2. Or examine the references section if you want to look up the actual studies.

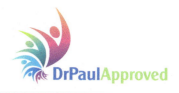

BUILDING NATURAL IMMUNITY

Please realize that, long term, you want to have immunity to COVID-19. This virus is now a part of our lives and those who develop immunity will survive it just as we have survived hundreds if not thousands of viruses in our lives. The question is this: what is the best way to get lasting immunity?

A look at history tells us that natural immunity is far more robust and lasting than that acquired from a vaccine. Since there is no vaccine AND the vaccines that are being worked on are being rushed to market without any long-term safety testing, my vote is that we develop a test to determine who needs the vaccine and only vaccinate the high-risk individuals who did not get natural immunity. That way we allow the young and healthy adults who seem to do just fine with COVID-19 develop natural herd immunity for the rest of us.

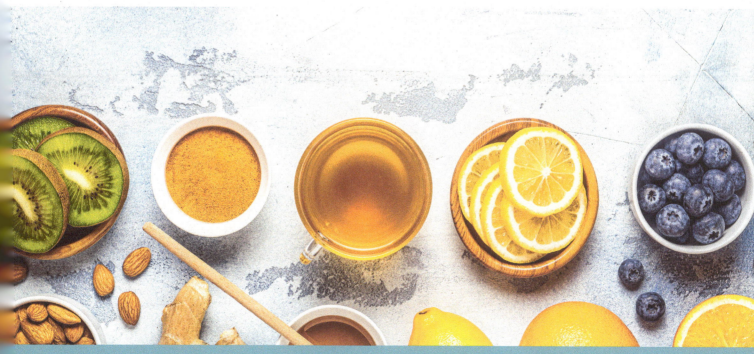

The information in this book is educational and Informational only: IT IS NOT MEDICAL ADVICE. It is not intended to diagnose or treat. No pharmaceutical or dietary supplement has been proven in long-term placebo-controlled studies to treat or prevent COVID-19.

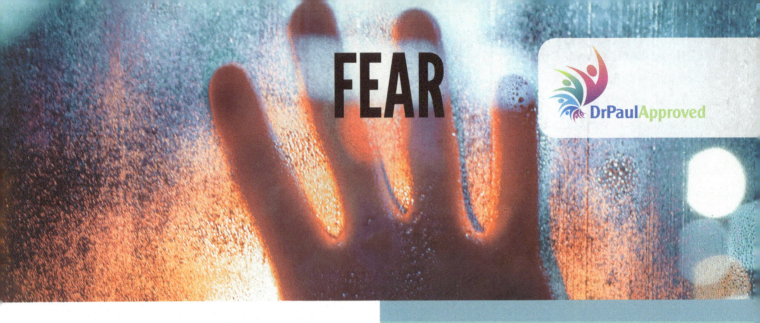

FEAR

DrPaulApproved

Why are people afraid?

Basically, because we are hearing an endless drum beat of bad news, data that is distorted and near worthless advice if you are infected: "Call your doctor, but don't go in to see him or her or go to the hospital." I say near worthless because I am one of those doctors. My team and I care for over 15,000 patients, and with COVID-19 we are wanting to keep these patients away from others for obvious reasons yet still provide care if they really need it. Many offices have just gone virtual, and are not seeing patients at all.

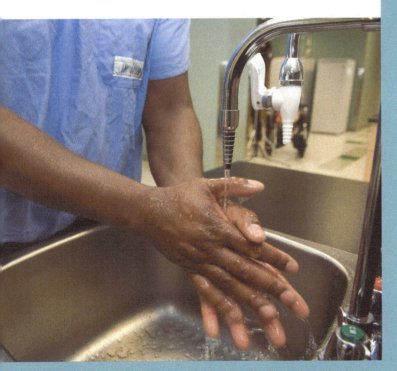

If we feel like we have control over a situation, we are less likely to feel afraid. Knowing that we can do some things to reduce the risk of developing COVID-19, may at least minimize some of the fear. That's why you need to do everything in your ability to avoid infection:

1. Wash your hands with soap and water after each time you touch anything someone else may have touched.
2. Practice social distancing especially if you are sick or someone you must be around is not well. Quarantine yourself if you are ill or exposed to COVID-19.
3. If you happen to be older or at high risk due to underlying conditions you must absolutely stay isolated and only a healthy (unexposed) family should be in your home.
4. Reduce stress. Yes, turn off that news.
5. Eat real fruits and vegetables.
6. Get some exercise and if they will let you – get outside and get some sunshine (not sunburn). Take supplements known to boost the immune system. I will discuss some of these later in the book. Practice mindfulness, do something for someone else and double your efforts to improve your physical, emotional and spiritual well-being.

The information in this book is educational and Informational only: IT IS NOT MEDICAL ADVICE. It is not intended to diagnose or treat. No pharmaceutical or dietary supplement has been proven in long-term placebo-controlled studies to treat or prevent COVID-19.

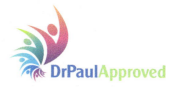

I don't want you to end up like my friend Bud. He is not allowed any visitors—not even his wife.

"What are they doing for you," I asked him?

"Nothing yet!"

He was already on oxygen and now they were just waiting for him to need intubation for respiratory support if the pneumonia progresses. What a terrible situation that in your time of greatest need you can't even have your loved ones near you! No one can visit. I can't help him and no one will be able to help you if you let this get bad enough that you need to be hospitalized.

Don't wait to do what you need to do until you are going to the ER or hospital. Once in that system you may end up in lockdown isolation with no access to the potentially life-saving supplements and treatments I'll be sharing with you.

What is the establishment telling you to do if sick? Call your doctor, but in many cases, they won't see you. Go to the emergency room where you likely will be triaged outside the hospital and sent home unless you are near needing oxygen support. Once in the hospital it is total isolation and they wait for you to need oxygen, then intubation and ventilation and hope you are not going to die. In places like New York, with ventilators in short supply, doctors may now even have to make the horrific decision which patients to treat and which to let die without treatment.

Pharmaceutical companies are rushing to find anything that might help. The latest, and worth a try for sure, is the malaria drug chloroquine. While this is being touted by some leaders as a solution, the truth, as stated clearly by Dr Antoni Fauci (White House Coronavirus Task Force and Medical Director of the National Institute of Allergy and Infectious Disease) "there is anecdotal evidence that the malaria drug chloroquine may help" but he went on to say "today (March 21, 2020) there are no proven safe and effective treatments for coronavirus."

Given the lack of safe and effective treatments from the pharmaceutical industry, it seems wise and prudent to look at safe approaches that are known to boost the immune system from the world of supplements and integrative medicine!

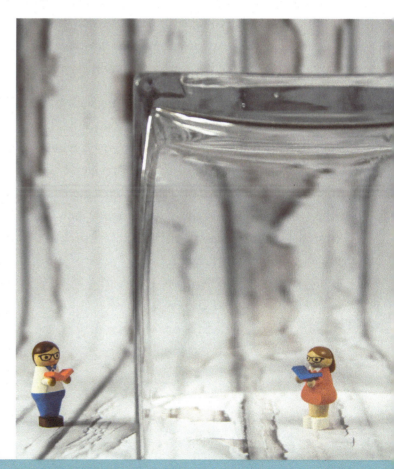

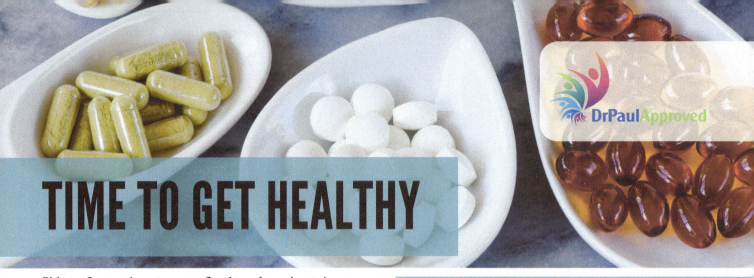

TIME TO GET HEALTHY

I'd say for too long many of us have been ignoring lifestyle choices, our dietary habits and have basically ignored the fact that we and we alone are responsible for how healthy our body is. We alone choose what food we put in our mouths. The exception here is those without the financial means or the availability of healthy food choices. We alone choose every day whether or not we are moving and exercising more or less. We choose to engage in stressful activities or refuse to turn off the news or put down the screen that keeps our stress level maxed out. We have allowed ourselves to become addicted or dependent on drugs or alcohol or nicotine or any number of substances or behaviors that are not boosting our immune systems.

We alone refuse to take immune-boosting supplements and we choose to listen to the pharmaceutical-funded mainstream medicine doctors, government and the media who ignore all the peer-reviewed articles that show benefits of dietary supplements while broadcasting loud and clear any study, however insignificant it may have been, that shows a problem with a vitamin or supplement.

WHAT DOES AN ANTI-INFLAMMATORY DIET DO?

Your immune system becomes activated when your body recognizes anything that is foreign—such as an invading microbe, plant pollen, or chemical. This can trigger inflammation. We need inflammation in the beginning of an infection as this helps us fight the invader. When patients with COVID-19 are struggling to breathe, the inflammation that was their friend is out of control and is causing more harm than good. Although the key supplements I am sharing can optimize your immune system and keep inflammation balanced, don't forget that what you eat is the most powerful tool you have.

Avoid these foods that tend to cause inflammation:
- Baked goods using refined flour, and most processed foods high in carbohydrates
- Sugar and soda
- Processed meats (deli, hot dogs, sausage), fatty red meat
- Partially hydrogenated fats (margarine, shortening)

Immune-boosting foods that don't stoke the wrong kind of inflammation are:
- Green leafy vegetables
- Fatty fish like salmon, mackerel, sardines Olive oil
- Berries, citrus (most fruits)

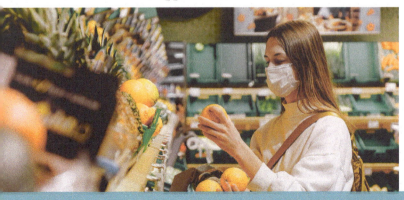

The information in this book is educational and Informational only: IT IS NOT MEDICAL ADVICE. It is not intended to diagnose or treat. No pharmaceutical or dietary supplement has been proven in long-term placebo-controlled studies to treat or prevent COVID-19.

TAKING YOUR HEALTH INTO YOUR OWN HANDS IS EMPOWERING

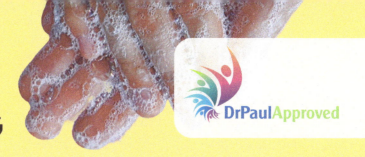

I'm going to empower you with the information you need to survive and navigate this crisis with confidence. That said, please know that the ideas here have been tested with my family, my friends and many patients but are not extensively published in peer-reviewed publications.

I first learned about Argentyn 23 solution several years ago at a MAPS (Medical Academy of Pediatric Special Needs) conference. I approached the booth in the vendors' area and the representative for this company was excited out of his mind to share his information with me because I was so skeptical AND I had life-long sinus infections. "You're my favorite kind of customer because I can show you how effective this stuff is," he said. He shared some of the science, how these are the finest silver particles available and how they have an antibacterial and antiviral effect. "Take these and spray a couple times on each nostril several times a day today and come see me tomorrow." I was remarkably better within a day and have only needed antibiotics once in the past few years. This is from a guy who lived on antibiotics half the time for his whole adult life and indeed struggled with sinus infections as a child. I even had sinus surgery a decade ago which helped for about 6 months!

I first learned about nebulizing Argentyn 23 a few months ago. I had diagnosed a patient with severe respiratory syncytial virus bronchiolitis and he had returned a few days later symptom free. "What happened, how did Johnny recover so fast?" I asked. His mom then told me about Argentyn 23 in the nebulizer. It had worked very quickly with rapid improvement in a day. This was the first time I had heard of this idea of nebulizing colloidal silver for respiratory infections like pneumonia and wheezing.

I've since read numerous reports and had close to 100 patient reports of quick resolution, typically within a day or two. My own wife had been coughing for over 3 weeks this past January and just couldn't kick it. Once we tried the nebulized Argentyn 23 the recovery was fast. She had already had both influenza B in November and Influenza A in December so I suspect she may have actually had COVID-19, we just weren't testing yet. Several of my staff have also experienced rapid recovery from what seemed to be severe respiratory viral infections of the lung these past couple months.

What I am reporting here is called "hearsay." Some refer to these types of reports as anecdotal and it is true – these are not the ideal classic double-blinded, placebo-controlled studies that we would need to be sure that what we have seen was real. This is however the same level of research as Dr Fauci stated existed for the idea of using the malaria drug chloroquine for COVID-19 infections. When we are dealing with a novel virus as dangerous and potentially fatal as these COVID-19 coronavirus infections, in order to bring useful treatment to the masses in a compressed timeline we must begin with case reports and anecdotal evidence. This should be followed by clinical trials and then ultimately double-blinded, placebo-controlled trials.

China is doing these types of studies including the use of high-dose vitamin C (either by IV or frequent high-dose oral) and the results are very promising. The world would do well to get on board with treatments like these that are actually making a huge impact by significantly reducing mortality and resulting in many recovering from COVID-19. Could the mortality rates of China and Italy be lower if they had used high-dose vitamin C?

The information in this book is educational and Informational only: IT IS NOT MEDICAL ADVICE. It is not intended to diagnose or treat. No pharmaceutical or dietary supplement has been proven in long-term placebo-controlled studies to treat or prevent COVID-19.

Imagine doing the things I am suggesting in this book and potentially reducing your risk of dying to close to zero? We won't know for sure until enough people try it. By trying the suggestions in this book you might get some diarrhea from the high-dose vitamin C, or a little tired from the melatonin, or perhaps slight bowel changes from the SBI – but those are risks I would take in a heartbeat given the mortality numbers coming out of Italy.

I would say to you who are skeptical I know how you feel as I felt the same way. What I have come to find out, however, is that the interventions I'm suggesting represent the best approaches available to us today. There is little downside other than potential diarrhea with the high-dose vitamin C, possible slight fatigue if you take melatonin in the morning or daytime and if it doesn't work you would be out the money spent.

I happen to believe with absolute confidence that there is nothing more powerful right now to empower and enable you to avoid serious infection – and to recover if you do get infected with COVID-19 – than the suggestions I'm making here.

If you are sick, especially if you have a cough, fatigue and fever you might have COVID-19. Some people who have the disease suffer from extreme nausea and/or diarrhea. There seems to be involvement in the chest and potentially a heart-related complication from this infection, so consider any new severe symptoms to be possible evidence of COVID-19 – at least until the world pandemic slows to a trickle.

Chances are you don't have COVID-19, so don't panic. But precaution is vital just in case you are exposed to the virus.

So, what do you do to protect yourself and your loved ones? The list below is not everything you could do to boost your immune system, but represents what I feel are key steps everyone should take if they can. The second half of this book will get to the hard science with references.

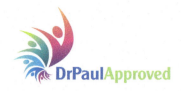

Avoid COVID-19 Exposure and Boost Your Immune System

1. Quarantine. Isolate yourself if you are high risk (older or with health issues).
2. Take Vitamin C 500 - 1,000 mg four times a day (lower dose if diarrhea).
3. Take melatonin 0.5 to 1 mg in am and 5 - 10 mg before bed.
4. Use colloidal silver* spray up each nostril and back of the throat twice a day. Start nebulizing 2 ml of these 4 times a day if you are coughing or having breathing issues.
5. Vitamin D + K2. Take 5,000 IU D3 daily.
6. SBI take 1 to 2.5 grams once or twice a day NAC (N-Acetyl cysteine) daily 250 - 1,000 mg a day (MitoCore is my favorite with lots more than just NAC. It has carnitine to give your cells energy and so much more).
7. CBD, if you can get the ultra-pure made from oranges CBD. Take 10 - 50 mg twice a day REDUCE STRESS. (reduce your time on devices, interact with positive people, meditate, volunteer, relax).
8. SLEEP. It is restorative, so guard your sleep as it is precious and vital.
9. EXERCISE. Do a little more than you have been (unless you already overdo).
10. WATER. Drink up to a gallon a day.
11. Share hope with your loved ones, friends and neighbors. Help someone every day.

WHERE TO PURCHASE THESE PRODUCTS?

Given the extreme magnitude of this pandemic, you may have to search before you find some of these supplements in stock. Get a link and enjoy my 25% professional discount. on most quality supplements on the market and be the first to get access to the bioidentical pure CBD here: click.drpaulapproved.com

The information in this book is educational and Informational only: IT IS NOT MEDICAL ADVICE. It is not intended to diagnose or treat. No pharmaceutical or dietary supplement has been proven in long-term placebo-controlled studies to treat or prevent COVID-19.

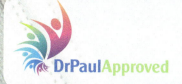

THE ANTIDOTE FOR FEAR

"The best antidote for fear is knowing what to do" from the astronauts on the international space station.

We are entering a phase of stress and uncertainty like nothing any of us have ever experienced.

Luck favors the prepared, and I want us to not only be prepared for ourselves but prepared so we can save the lives of our loved ones, our patients and as many who suffer in our community as possible.

The world, America, the city we live and work in and our families and friends will experience more disruption than we have ever experienced. Wuhan, China, South Korea, Italy and now much of Europe and the US are already experiencing a magnitude of suffering not seen since war times. Some of our acquaintances and perhaps even family or friends may die. I don't want that to happen, and I think we can drastically reduce those odds by taking a few vital steps.

A trip to any local grocer makes one thing clear; these are different times. There is no toilet paper to be found anywhere, and it is getting difficult to find vitamin C.

So how do we prepare?

Acknowledge that there are some unknowns here. I suspect I had this virus in December, but there is no way of knowing for sure until the antibody test becomes widely available. In January or February, my wife, kids and several of my employees had severe, hard to kick, coughs that were associated with horrible fatigue. I suspect they probably had COVID-19 also. I suspect many of you reading this who had the worst cough and fatigue (worst flu) of your lives may have had COVID-19. If it was COVID-19 then perhaps we've all been exposed and developed immunity. However, since we don't know, I want us to act as if we are all potentially vulnerable.

There is a definite age risk calculation to be made here.(4)

AGE	DEATH RATE
80+	14.8%
70-79	8.0%
60-69	3.6%
50-59	1.3%
40-49	0.4%
10-39	0.2%
0-9	0%

Something important to keep in mind: these numbers are based on total numbers of tests done, not the population exposed nor the number of sick people. In the USA we are so short of tests that the hospital I use the most, which is near my office, is turning away lots of sick people with cough and fever but who weren't "that sick," WITHOUT testing them as the hospital only had a limited supply of tests! Many of the tests they conducted could not be run due to lack of reagent.(5)

The information in this book is educational and Informational only: IT IS NOT MEDICAL ADVICE. It is not intended to diagnose or treat. No pharmaceutical or dietary supplement has been proven in long-term placebo-controlled studies to treat or prevent COVID-19.

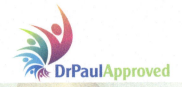

Given that we are truly only testing the sickest of the sick, my best wild guess is that you can reduce these fatality numbers by a factor of 100 to 1,000, which would make the death rate if exposed less than 1/10,000 to 1/100,000 for most of us. This virus is very contagious. I've seen projections that over half the country will be infected. We have 300 million people in the USA. If we end up with 15,000 deaths out of the 150 million infected that would be a death rate of 1/100,000.

The number of people in the USA dying from COVID-19 may end up being grossly inflated by the process of making COVID-19 the cause of death when other reasons existed. We learned that 99% of those who died in Italy had at least one underlying condition. We will only know the real impact on total mortality when we see total mortality numbers for each country compared to that of the previous decade. If we are merely substituting COVID-19 where in previous years the cause of death would have been influenza or heart disease, we would realize that the total effect of this pandemic has been grossly exaggerated.

There are still going to be huge numbers released, more and more every day for the next month or two and maybe longer, as we are going to start to do more testing. The drastic quarantines (probably a good idea) will flatten the curve, meaning this will go on longer than it did in China. As we test more, we will get more positives, so not only are the growing numbers of infected real, but the numbers will seem enormous as we are now catching up with our testing. People who are recovering will be included and people with mild symptoms or none at all will be included in the numbers once we start testing everyone.

Now the Good News

I think we can reduce our risk to near ZERO by taking some concrete steps now!

We can absolutely boost our immune systems so that we fight this virus off. Don't wait any longer – please. I'm writing a book as fast as I can so everyone that is interested in actually doing something to prevent and or treat the infection has some concrete things they can do. I've outlined above many of the key steps as I wanted them near the beginning so readers could get right to the key information fast. Most of us in the world don't even have a week or two to waste thinking about this and what to do. This situation requires ACTION. And NOW!

Prevention-Keys to Avoid Getting COVID-19

Treat every surface you touch as potentially contaminated with the virus and wash your hands after touching anything that might have been touched by someone else. This COVID-19 infection is primarily transmitted by breathing the air that an infected person just coughed or sneezed into, or more than likely you touched a surface that has been touched by an infected person. After touching an infected surface, you touch your face, rub your nose and BAM – you are infected.

I am not afraid because I know what to do to minimize getting infected and I know what to do if I do get infected! That is why I'm sharing this with you, so you too can go forward with confidence, knowledge and a plan. I'm also in one of the highest risk groups: medical professionals who see sick patients. And I'm male and over 60 years old. I'm still not afraid. Not careless, not reckless but cautiously optimistic that I have a healthy immune system that can handle this virus, AND I'll be as careful as possible within reason.

The information in this book is educational and Informational only: IT IS NOT MEDICAL ADVICE. It is not intended to diagnose or treat. No pharmaceutical or dietary supplement has been proven in long-term placebo-controlled studies to treat or prevent COVID-19.

What do I mean by being as careful as possible within reason?

Health care professionals are on the front lines of this war on COVID-19. The respiratory therapists and intensive care doctors and those working to keep patients from needing a ventilator are the front line. We've already seen that lack of equipment has increased risks for those on the front line. While in the beginning it made sense to send any medical provider who may have been exposed home, we have quickly realized that doing this would result in no medical providers being available in very short order. To my colleagues: please consider the immune-boosting suggestions I am making here. Our patients need us now more than ever!

Those of us who are immunocompromised or older or you just don't feel you can take the risk of working in a medical setting, or perhaps where you work there are just too many people in closed spaces – it is absolutely OK that you take time off. Self-quarantine makes sense. If you have a loved one you live with or must visit regularly who is at very high risk, it makes sense not to go to work or be around others at a time when the COVID-19 epidemic is raging and we have limited data. Be thinking about your plan when this gets way worse and people in your town are dying. I'm planning to be part of the solution and to help as many as I can, and maybe you can too.

Make sure your loved ones and friends and co-workers know that there are options, but don't pressure anyone. Most people are afraid of alternative approaches and the media is frequently making unsubstantiated warnings about unproven remedies. I'll agree that the proof is not at the level of well-controlled, double-blinded, placebo-controlled studies, but that doesn't mean there is no evidence for the recommendations I am making here.

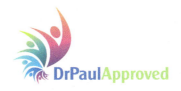

If you care about someone, you should be sharing this with your loved ones, friends and acquaintances. You will want each of your contacts to make decisions for themselves. Please feel free to share this book with anyone you care about. We do need a wartime mentality going forward. This will be a time where many are panicking, and most will be living in fear.

Wash your hands every time you touch something that someone else has touched. This gets complicated with doorknobs at work, but perhaps carry wipes, gloves or at the very least be very careful to wipe down everything you touch and wash your hands the minute you can. It is especially important to avoid touching your face. Certainly, before and after each encounter wash your hands and wipe off things you have touched.

Wear a mask when seeing patients with cough or fever or flu-like symptoms, chest pain, shortness of breath, nausea or diarrhea. A bandana is better than nothing if you don't have a mask. This is not a requirement but a suggestion. Given shortages of masks at the time of this writing, use your same mask for as much of the day as you can. CDC says bandanas work and the COVID-19 is actually a very large particle so I support that. At my office, Integrative Pediatrics, because of how we look with the masks on, I've suggested we call ourselves the Integrative Bandits, saving the children, our friends and their families. The masks provide Safer Passage in a world gone crazy with a novel virus that IS TREATABLE and PREVENTABLE.

Let me be clear that I am not guaranteeing every patient will get well and every infection will be prevented, but in general the measures I'm recommending can reduce risk significantly.

The information in this book is educational and Informational only: IT IS NOT MEDICAL ADVICE. It is not intended to diagnose or treat. No pharmaceutical or dietary supplement has been proven in long-term placebo-controlled studies to treat or prevent COVID-19.

BOOST YOUR IMMUNE SYSTEM

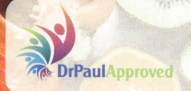

I mentioned earlier in this book some lifestyle strategies and dietary supplements that can be used to boost your immunity. Here, I'm going to let you know more about why I'm recommending these strategies and supplements.

Eat healthy real foods (lots of fresh fruits and vegetables). Reduce stress. Don't sit and watch the news for hours – someone will tell you the important stuff, or check in for 15 minutes once a day on your favorite news channel. I can tell you right now what the news will say. The number of infected and dead is going up!

If you have health impairing habits, now is the time to say goodbye to them: for example, smoking, excessive eating, drinking or drug use, too much time watching TV or staying bent over your electronic devices, to name a few obvious ones.

Take Vitamin C 1,000 mg 4 - 6 times a day if your bowels can tolerate it. If you end up with diarrhea or other digestive complaints from too much vitamin C, reduce the dose but still take it frequently if you can tolerate it. I'm repeating myself here – but I truly think you need to understand that for this virus at this time, high-dose frequent vitamin C is probably the most important thing you can do. I wish those designing trials of pharmaceutical drugs for this virus would have a high-dose vitamin C arm to their studies. Vitamin C is a powerful antioxidant and one that humans have lost the capacity to make for ourselves. We have to eat or drink it.

Take Melatonin (0.5 to 1 mg in the morning and at noon and 5 - 10 mg before bed). Melatonin has been used successfully to assist with sleep.

We know that melatonin levels are very low in newborns but quickly rise such that children under age 9 have the highest levels. Levels then drop progressively as we age such that the very old have extremely low levels. This may explain, in part, why children seem to be relatively protected from COVID-19 and the very old are at such high risk. Melatonin is an antioxidant which helps us fight infections.

Drink lots of water. Adults should set a goal to drink a gallon a day.

Exercise in moderation – just start walking outdoors (yup outdoors - unless it has become unlawful to do so). Exercise not only boosts our natural endorphins but is good for blood flow and if you get a sweat you are eliminating toxins from the body, an added benefit. The overall "runners-high" that many experience is a real thing that occurs due to that boost of endorphins. After exercise in moderation, you will find that the soreness you may have passes. It's a different soreness than the deep fatigue of the flu or COVID-19.

NAC (N-acetyl cysteine) boosts the all-important antioxidant glutathione. There are preparations of liposomal glutathione that might be worth a try. However, glutathione is a molecule that oxidizes very easily and oxidized glutathione is worse for you than doing nothing! For this reason I prefer that you take some NAC and let your body make the glutathione it needs. NAC tastes horrible – like rotten eggs – so it is very difficult to get into a powder or solution that tastes okay. Those who can take NAC in capsule form by all means do so at a usual dose of 250 - 600 mg for adults. I've seen doses of up to 1,000 mg recommended for COVID-19 infections.

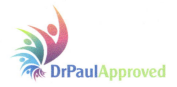

MitoCORE (made by Ortho Molecular Products) – One to 2 capsules twice a day or ¼ to half a scoop twice a day not only provides the NAC but also carnitine to give your cells energy and a host of other immune-boosting vitamins and the right methylated B vitamins. Methylation is a process where the body converts the damaging amino acid homocysteine into the essential amino acid methionine and the non-essential amino acid cysteine.

SBI (Serum Bovine immunoglobulin) – May bind coronavirus in the gut (half a scoop daily or a little bit twice a day). It also just came out in capsules. While the powder is relatively tasteless it does clump easily and can be difficult to get into solution. I use an eggbeater which works just fine, other than a little foam. SBI has plenty of research around its ability to bind toxins in the gut. Coronaviruses have an affinity for the gut,(3) so this seems like a wise move to help bind it and rid the body before it enters the body, or at least to usher it out in the stool.

CBD (I prefer the new CBD made from oranges that is soon to be available). Take 10 - 50 mg once or twice a day. If you are using products derived from hemp, perhaps use lower doses to avoid the THC and toxin exposures that may be causing more harm than good.

It may be prudent to avoid ibuprofen which may actually enhance binding of the coronavirus to the ACE receptors in the lungs. This is only theoretical at this time and the CDC and WHO do not believe ibuprofen increases your risk and that you can continue to take it if you have a medical condition that requires it. The journal Lancet published the hypothesis that SARS-CoV-2 binds to the epithelial cells of the lung, intestine, kidney, and blood vessels through angiotensin-converting enzyme 2 (ACE2).(6)

The expression of ACE2 is substantially increased in patients with hypertension and type 1 or type 2 diabetes, who are treated with ACE inhibitors and angiotensin II type-I receptor blockers (ARBs), which results in an upregulation of ACE2 potentially giving the virus greater entry into the body. ACE2 can also be increased by thiazolidinediones and ibuprofen.

As humans we are tribal or community-requiring animals. We don't do well in isolation. Call your loved ones who are at home and may be freaking out and share this advice so they too can reduce their stress levels and feel more empowered and prepared. Go for walks and meet your neighbors on the sidewalks or local parks if you are still allowed to use them. Remember that the greatest exposures will be indoors. Still honor social distancing, even when outside, but get outside as much as you can.

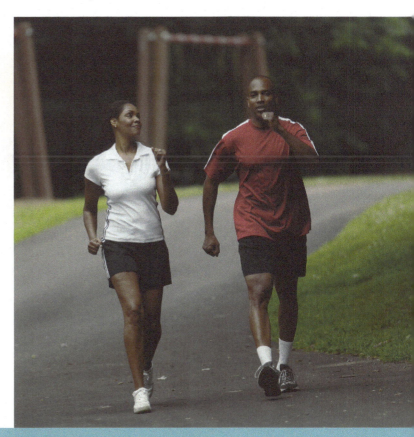

The information in this book is educational and Informational only: IT IS NOT MEDICAL ADVICE. It is not intended to diagnose or treat. No pharmaceutical or dietary supplement has been proven in long-term placebo-controlled studies to treat or prevent COVID-19.

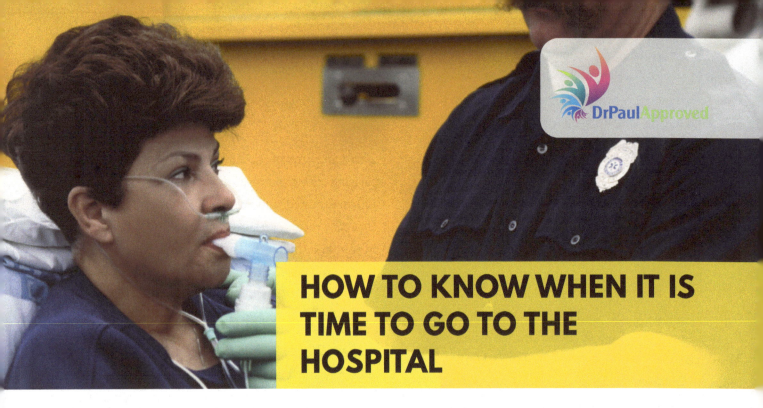

HOW TO KNOW WHEN IT IS TIME TO GO TO THE HOSPITAL

If you really have COVID-19 and are starting to need oxygen, how would you know when to go to the hospital? Get a pulse oximeter while they are still available. These devices measure your oxygen levels. They are especially important for older people and individuals with an underlying condition. My advice is to stay away from the hospital unless your oxygen levels are dramatically low and you need a ventilator. Once you are at the hospital and if you have COVID-19 you will be in total isolation with no contact with your loved ones even if you are dying. It will be near impossible to do the alternative therapies that are likely the exact things that will enable your body to heal and prevent death on a ventilator from ARDS (Adult Respiratory Distress Syndrome).

The oxygen dissociation curve gets steep around an oxygen saturation of 90% or less. What that means is that as your oxygenation enters the 80's you could very quickly deteriorate, so you need to be near a hospital and you should consult your doctor or the best facility that could care for you in the event you need respiratory support. When oxygenation is around 90% or less you generally start to experience some air hunger.

You may find yourself taking occasional deep breaths – like a gasp. If you are starting to struggle for air, then it is indeed time to be evaluated, regardless of your pulse ox reading. Generally, if your pulse oximeter is reading over 90% breathing room air (meaning you are not requiring extra oxygen) you are probably still fine. While a pulse ox of 97%-100% is considered normal, some of these inexpensive meters are not as accurate. I recently had a pulse ox of 95% and this was after a very intense CrossFit workout while feeling totally healthy. I share that so you realize that how you are feeling is more important than a number on the pulse oximeter. When you feel short of breath AND your pulse ox is 90 or less you definitely need to be evaluated.

Of note, Bud shared that he had his oxygenation dropping below 80% at times, but he still refused intubation, preferring to struggle on. You see, once intubated, you are also sedated and as Bud put it "I wanted to be able to fight this thing".

The information in this book is educational and Informational only: IT IS NOT MEDICAL ADVICE. It is not intended to diagnose or treat. No pharmaceutical or dietary supplement has been proven in long-term placebo-controlled studies to treat or prevent COVID-19.

WHAT TO DO WHEN YOU HAVE A COVID-19 INFECTION

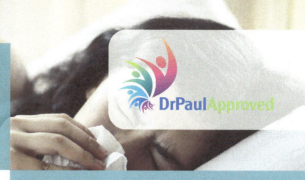

A lot of this I have covered in the section "Boost Your Immune System".

If I had worsening respiratory symptoms with impending oxygen requirement (pulse ox dropping below 90% on room air) or if I didn't have a pulse ox and needed to breathe faster and deeper and had a sensation of air hunger, then this is what I would do:

Homeopathic Colloidal Silver:

Consider nebulized Argentyn 23 several times a day. If Argentyn 23 is unavailable, then use Sovereign Silver. Nebulize 1 to 2 ml 4 times a day for mild symptoms and every 1 to 2 hours if your oxygen levels are dropping and you may be needing to go to the hospital soon. Generally, they won't do much for you at the hospital until your oxygen levels are around 90% or less. Some busy hospitals where they are short on ventilators are sending patients home with oxygen to buy a few more days. I actually would choose that option if offered and you have transportation back to the hospital if you get worse.

Portable nebulizers and the colloidal silver can be purchased online without a prescription. I prefer Argentyn 23, with next best being Sovereign Silver, but if these become unavailable and you are in trouble I would consider other brands. I just don't have any experience with them. Worst case scenario (when we are out of nebulizers); one could perhaps use an infuser or mist machine for the Argentyn 23 or silver solution and breathe it in from that! You would likely need to put more solution into it to make it work. These homeopathic silver solutions have a concentration generally between 10 and 30 ppm (parts per million), which is basically water, so I'm not worried about how much you nebulize, whether it is 2 ml or 30 ml. Cost would become the prohibitive factor.

Vitamin C:

Take Vitamin C at least 1,000 mg every 15 to 30 minutes while awake if you are having respiratory symptoms and may have COVID-19. The only limit to how much you can take is how much you can tolerate before getting severe diarrhea. There are reports of using up to 50,000 mg of vitamin C for those struggling with COVID-19 lung infections. Nobel prize winner the late Linus Pauling was a strong advocate for high-dose vitamin C and is reported to have been taking about 10,000 mg daily for much of his adult life. That was just to maintain health, so the safety of high-dose vitamin C is not in question, as long as you don't get dehydration from diarrhea.

Melatonin:

Melatonin use for COVID-19 infections addresses inflammation, acts as an antioxidant, and regulates the immune response. Melatonin has a great safety profile. While the evidence of melatonin's potential benefits for COVID-19 infections is unclear, its use in experimental animal models and in studies on humans has shown efficacy and safety. One could predict that melatonin use by COVID-19 patients would be highly beneficial.(7) If you are infected with COVID-19, take melatonin 0.5 mg a few times during the day, although it may make you tired. If diabetic, watch your blood sugar and insulin needs, and take 10 - 20 mg before bed.

The information in this book is educational and Informational only: IT IS NOT MEDICAL ADVICE. It is not intended to diagnose or treat. No pharmaceutical or dietary supplement has been proven in long-term placebo-controlled studies to treat or prevent COVID-19.

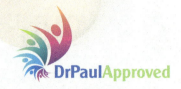

CBD:

CBD (cannabidiol) balances the immune system, but more importantly is known to increase the number of natural killer (NK) cells.(8) These NK cells act like soldiers that go after and kill unwanted invaders in the body. I'll discuss this property of CBD more later in my book. While CBD was not specifically tested against COVID-19, it would be reasonable to think that CBD may help boost the natural abilities of the body to fight this infection. (NOT A MEDICAL CLAIM no pharmaceuticals or supplements have had long-term placebo-controlled testing against this new virus).

NAC, MitoCobre, SBI:

NAC boosts glutathione, perhaps the most important antioxidant molecule that also helps fight infections. MitoCORE is a product in powder or capsule that has a perfect combination of NAC with carnitine and other key nutrients to boost your immune system and enhance mitochondrial function and cellular energy. Your mitochondria are the powerhouses of your cells. The extreme fatigue described by those with the more severe COVID-19 infections is a signal that the cells are stressed and could use more energy. SBI, (Serum Bovine Immunoglobulin) binds endotoxins in the gut helping usher them out of the body and in so doing also protecting the gut immune system (GALT - Gut Associated Lymphoid Tissue).

Caution

Don't be confused or dissuaded by the talking heads on TV who are fast to warn you of frauds and "bogus" medical treatments. I've heard the examples of vitamin C and colloidal silver used as examples of these "bogus" or "fraudulent" treatments being peddled for profit. You can bet that if it doesn't profit big pharma then the media that is bought and paid for by big pharma will try to discourage you from trying it. Don't feel any obligation to purchase anything from anywhere. I share my resources because I'm asked all the time "what do you use, Dr. Paul?" and "Where do you get it?"

You will undoubtedly hear that these natural remedies are unproven, untested, and even dangerous and to beware of those unscrupulous, unethical doctors and charlatans trying to profit from you. In the next breath they will tell you there is nothing you can do, but pharmaceutical companies are fast-tracking vaccines and medicines that will soon be available. In the meantime stay home and good luck. There is nothing you can do but wait.

Really?

Would you let your loved one die when a potentially helpful approach that is harmless is at the corner store or vitamin shop or a click away online?

Remember: we are in this together. I don't want anyone to die on my watch, which could happen if you go to the hospital without doing all these things. Unfortunately, once in the hospital you aren't allowed to bring in anything from the outside AND they are severely limiting visitors, probably to zero if you are positive for COVID-19.

I am not in the least bit afraid because I have the tools I have mentioned here. And I don't want you to be afraid either.

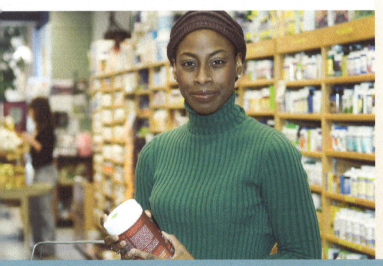

The information in this book is educational and Informational only: IT IS NOT MEDICAL ADVICE. It is not intended to diagnose or treat. No pharmaceutical or dietary supplement has been proven in long-term placebo-controlled studies to treat or prevent COVID-19.

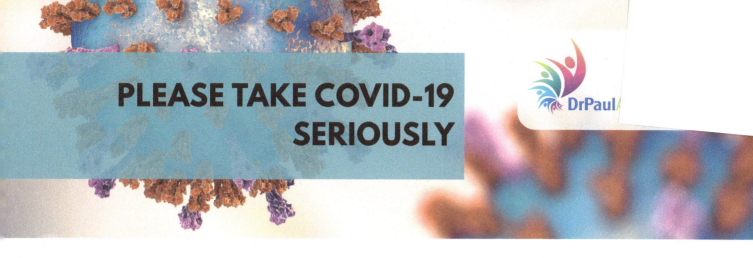

PLEASE TAKE COVID-19 SERIOUSLY

Even though we should not be afraid, this virus is for real. It may be 1,000 times more infectious at the level of the lungs than SARS and MERS,(3) so until we get through the storm that is coming, be prepared. It will infect more people as the R0 rate (the number of people an infected person will infect) is being reported as 2.3 as compared to a 1.3 R0 rate for the flu. And, once infected with COVID-19 it appears to be especially damaging to the lungs.

How seasonal flu and COVID-19 compare	FLU	COVID-19
R0 number Estimate of many people you will infect	1.3	2.3
Incubation (days)	1-4	1-14
Hospitalization rate	2%	19%
Case fatality rate	0.1%	1-3.4%

[modified from WHO, CDC NCBI data]

It is clear that COVID-19 is more contagious, generally has a longer incubation time meaning those infected can have no symptoms for up to 14 days, has a hospitalization rate of 19% compared to the 2% we see with influenza, and the apparent fatality rate appears to be over 1%, which is at least 10 times that of the flu. These numbers however, are inflated by the fact that only the sickest are getting tested, as well as people who come in close contact with them.

Most children under 10 will be fine. Just as we see each year that some children die from the flu, there has already been a report of an infant dying from COVID-19, and there will be more. We generally learn later that these were children with significant underlying health issues so for healthy children I still feel confident that COVID-19 does not pose a major threat. I wish we could find a way to have COVID-19 parties for them but alas that would not work as they would take it home to someone at risk and, well, you can see how that would not go well. No! I am NOT advocating COVID-19 parties!

Comparisons with the flu are problematic because for years the CDC and our news media who repeat everything that comes out from the CDC, have lumped flu death statistics together with bacterial pneumonia deaths as if these were "flu" deaths.

Why?

One can only speculate as to why such a massive intentional distortion of the truth would be perpetrated on our public. My best guess: it is to create fear. Fear of the flu will lead you to get your flu shot. With almost half the country now getting flu shots each year in a country with about 300 million people that is a lot of flu shots. A lot of money for a vaccine that is not very effective, if effective at all.

The information in this book is educational and Informational only: IT IS NOT MEDICAL ADVICE. It is not intended to diagnose or treat. No pharmaceutical or dietary supplement has been proven in long-term placebo-controlled studies to treat or prevent COVID-19.

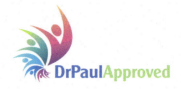

Here are the real numbers as presented by the American Lung Association.(9) In 2010 there were more than one million hospitalizations due to pneumonia with only an additional 7,000 being due to influenza "with influenza rates generally too low to allow for meaningful comparison."

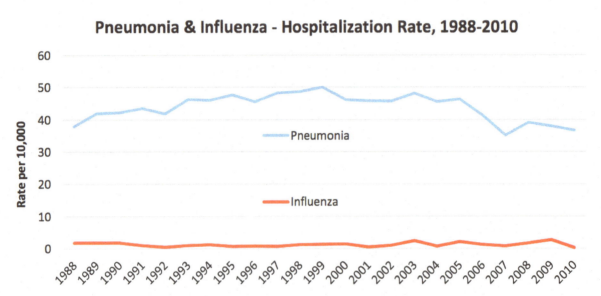

You can see that even just counting hospitalizations, influenza is relatively insignificant. And we aren't even talking about deaths here which clearly would be almost entirely due to pneumonia of other causes and not influenza. You can see that the influenza vaccine program has basically done little if anything to change the hospitalization rates in the USA.

Our leaders at the CDC and WHO are heading toward repeating the same distortion but this time instead of calling all deaths "the flu" doctors are being guided to label the cause of death "COVID-19", even in cases where this has not been proven or when there are underlying causes that may actually be the main reason the person died.

From the CDC website: "Coronavirus disease deaths are identified using the ICD–10 code U07.1. Deaths are coded to U07.1 when coronavirus disease 2019 or COVID-19 are reported as a cause that contributed to death on the death certificate. These can include laboratory confirmed cases, as well as cases without laboratory confirmation.

When they roll out vaccines for COVID-19, they will be rushed to market, with no long-term safety trials and no liability for those who make them. If you have allowed fear to take over, you may well be willing to roll your sleeve up and become part of the next vaccine experiment on a massive level.

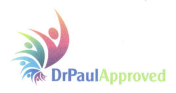

Please share this information with all the people you know and care about. We will look back and remember 2020 as perhaps the most difficult year of our lives. I want us to look back and smile knowing we did everything we could to be prepared, to be healthy and to help those less fortunate than we were.

When you know better you do better.

There will be some who just cannot accept alternative or complementary medicine approaches. I have many family members in that category. I'm just praying they make it through these difficult times given their contempt and rejection of these simple suggestions. We have been so brainwashed into believing everything we hear on the news, from the CDC, from our elected officials, from the wonderful pharmaceutical industry that wants you to know they are working diligently to come up with cures and vaccines.

Those unwilling or unable to learn in times like these may perish. Some undoubtedly will suffer as a result of their choice not to be open minded. Contempt prior to investigation I would say.

I'm asked: how can I share all this when I will be looked upon by the establishment as a Quack?

My response is simple. If I know something that can save lives – lots of lives – and I make the decision to keep that information to myself, well, that is horrible and I then become part of the problem. If I witness an injustice that I know how to make better, and do nothing, then I am also a perpetrator.

What about you?

Will you do what it takes for your family?

Would you risk ridicule to at least make sure your loved ones have potentially lifesaving information?

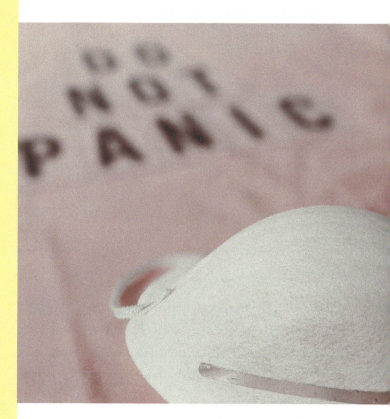

We are at war. The enemy is as much fear as it is the virus, especially when there are simple potentially life-saving strategies that I have outlined.

Please share this with everyone who is open minded and willing to learn, willing to be empowered and willing to take control of their lives.

There will be a push by the mainstream to discredit alternative approaches – it is already happening. They want the solution to be pharma driven and of course the vaccine rush is on!

Knowledge is power.

You are now POWERFUL!

Together we can get through this.

The information in this book is educational and Informational only: IT IS NOT MEDICAL ADVICE. It is not intended to diagnose or treat. No pharmaceutical or dietary supplement has been proven in long-term placebo-controlled studies to treat or prevent COVID-19.

WORKING TOGETHER IN COMMUNITY

This is a viral pandemic, and not the kind of war or natural disaster that totally disrupts our food supply and ability to shop and purchase basic needs. There will be shortages that are temporary due to particular factories or industries being shut down for a few months, but we will all get through this.

Therefore, there is no need to hoard goods. Supply chains remain open so If we refrain from hoarding, everyone will be able to get what they need, when they need it.

Take advantage of special hours for vulnerable populations like the elderly if they are available and you qualify. We all should be doing all we can not to expose those who are very old, medically fragile or with underlying health conditions that put them at greater risk.

Social distancing is critical any time we are indoors with strangers, like shopping or going to the office. In many states the orders are to "stay at home" unless you are engaged in essential activities. Grocery shopping is of course an essential activity but limit your contact with others and if you have higher risk individuals try to have them stay at home and not venture into the grocery stores and shopping areas. The guideline to allow 6 feet of distance between you, your fellow customers, and grocery store employees is often impossible to follow in the stores but give it your best shot!

Remember that anything someone else has touched from grocery carts or grocery bags could have a virus on it. No need to panic – just avoid touching your face and wash your hands with soap and water as soon as you can. And wipe down everything you touched before washing your hands.

If you work in places where exposures are likely, or after shopping or visiting the doctor's office or being on mass transit or other indoor spaces, consider stripping your clothes right into the washer when you get home.

Some of these suggestions feel over the top, and may indeed be so, but for parts of the world where we are still experiencing a wave of new cases and deaths, caution is wise.

Here is the sequence of events for the towns that are deep into this already, as tweeted March 9th, 2020 by Jason VanSchoor, shared by an intensivist in Northern Italy:

"At first there are a few positive cases, and mild measures are taken, people are told to avoid emergency departments but still hang out in groups, everyone says not to panic. Then some people start developing moderate resp failures and a few severe ones that need to be intubated, but most are avoiding the emergency rooms so everything looks great. Next tons of patients develop moderate resp failure, overwhelming the ICU's with staff becoming overworked and sick themselves. As things deteriorate OR's (operating rooms) and every location that has oxygen is being used. As staff get sick it gets difficult to cover for shifts, mortality spikes not only from the covid-19 infections but from all other causes that can't be treated properly."

The information in this book is educational and Informational only: IT IS NOT MEDICAL ADVICE. It is not intended to diagnose or treat. No pharmaceutical or dietary supplement has been proven in long-term placebo-controlled studies to treat or prevent COVID-19.

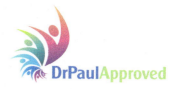

I can't stress enough the importance of being prepared for this. Think of the airline coming in for a crash landing and airbags are deployed. You put your mask on first so you can help others.

Are you prepared? Do you have your Respiratory Rescue Kit with at least one to spare in case you need to save another family member or friend?

Respiratory Rescue Kit

Nebulizer (portable or any kind you can get)

Argentyn 23 (or Sovereign Silver – if these are available, any kind you can get)

Pulse oximeter (this is nice to have to monitor your progress or need for oxygen)

911 Coronavirus Infection Kit

- Vitamin C (get enough to take the typical dose I mentioned previously every 30 minutes while awake)
- Melatonin (A low dose 0.5 – 1 mg during the day and 5 – 10 mg for before bed)
- Helpful:
  - SBI (Serum Bovine Immunoglobulin), or Enteragam.
  - MitoCORE by Ortho Molecular Products or another source of NAC
  - A good multivitamin
  - CBD

Are you calling your family and friends? If they aren't prepared, will you be helping them when they need help? Did you get an extra Respiratory Kit and Coronavirus Infection Kit for them?

Call them and do it now and as often as you or they need or want. Staying connected is an important part of the healing journey.

Be Prepared.

If you are not afraid at all then you are either very prepared or you have a combination of recklessness and faith beyond measure or a wish to die. You also might know that you have a robust healthy immune system due to meticulous self care, proper nutrition and you have done everything along the way that promotes a healthy immune system. I don't want you to be afraid. You don't need to be, as long as you are prepared. As I was reaching out to help Bud (he was still in the hospital on oxygen and his wife sick at home, both in quarantine), I became aware that there won't be enough nebulizers and Argentyn 23, vitamin C and melatonin to go around if this indeed infects 50% of the population.

I don't want you to hoard, as we are all in this together, but do plan for your family and loved ones, and if you have the means, plan for a few others to whom you might be a rescuing angel.

The information in this book is educational and Informational only: IT IS NOT MEDICAL ADVICE. It is not intended to diagnose or treat. No pharmaceutical or dietary supplement has been proven in long-term placebo-controlled studies to treat or prevent COVID-19.

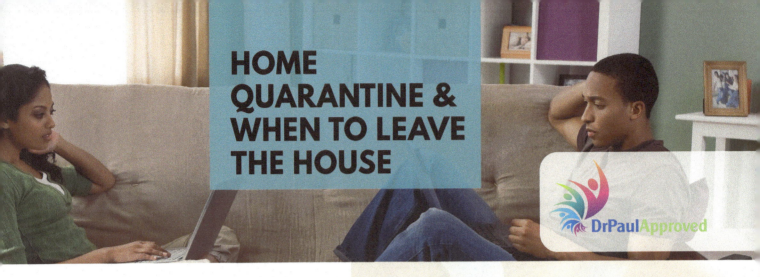

HOME QUARANTINE & WHEN TO LEAVE THE HOUSE

Those who are infected with COVID-19 are told to stay home and not leave the house. The question that follows is this: When is it OK to leave the house, for that quarantine to end? Each State or government may have their own policy, the CDC guidelines may change and your doctor may have the ability to guide you on this.

In Oregon, USA where I live and practice medicine, the Oregon Health Authority (OHA) gives us these guidelines.

If you aren't able to obtain a test to determine whether you still have COVID-19, you can stop isolating at home after you've met all three of these criteria:

1. Your fever has been gone for at least 72 hours (3 full days) without using medicines that reduce fevers.
2. Your other symptoms (for example, cough or shortness of breath) are gone.
3. At least a week has passed since your first developed symptoms appeared.

Your decision whether or not to leave your house should be made together with your doctor and state and local health departments, according to CDC guidelines.

ENCOURAGING NEWS FOR THE ELDERLY

This COVID-19 disease certainly seems to be more fatal for the elderly. This tends to instill fear in those older and their family members. My mom and dad both live in different retirement communities that are on lock-down. The death rate from the Kirkland Washington Care facility was horrible with about 35 deaths reported linked to COVID-19 in a population that was about 120 elderly before the outbreak began. That would be a death rate of one out of 3.4 residents or 29%. This was how this began in America. What seems to have happened there was that workers who are ill, continued to work not realizing this was more than just a common cold or the flu.

We've had a similar situation here in Oregon where the Oregon Veterans Home in Lebanon started having numerous cases of COVID-19. The good news now is that 13 of the 16 confirmed cases of COVID-19 at the Oregon Veterans' Home in Lebanon have recovered and there have only been 3 deaths from a total of 18 identified COVID-19 cases. That means of those infected only 1 of 6 have died or 16%. Since I don't have the total number of residents I cannot give the real risk which would be much lower than that.

The home's oldest resident, a World War II veteran who celebrated his 104th birthday with a small group of family this week, survived!

Now onto the science.

The information in this book is educational and Informational only: IT IS NOT MEDICAL ADVICE. It is not intended to diagnose or treat. No pharmaceutical or dietary supplement has been proven in long-term placebo-controlled studies to treat or prevent COVID-19.

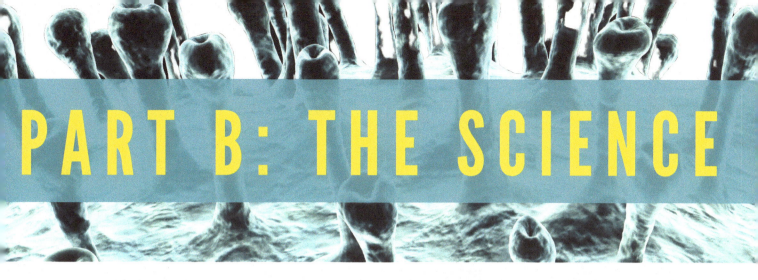

PART B: THE SCIENCE

The Virus

The SARS-CoV-2, novel coronavirus responsible for COVID-19 infection, is now taking over the entire world and is clearly the worst infectious pandemic the world has seen in a century. It can induce pneumonia in adult patients regardless of age and evidence is growing that it can cause pneumonia in children too, especially if they have underlying conditions.

Coronaviruses are a large family of viruses, with only a few known to cause disease in humans. Most coronaviruses infect animals, and a few have evolved to infect humans. SARS-CoV-2 clearly can infect humans and while it is thought to have started in bats this virus can easily spread from human to human making this one perhaps the most contagious coronavirus we have ever seen.

The WHO-China Joint Mission on Coronavirus Disease 2019 (COVID-19) report released February 28th 2020 gave us specific details of this virus.

On December 30th 2019, bronchoalveolar lavage samples were positive for pan-Betacoronavirus. "Using Illumina and nanopore sequencing, ...showed the closest relationship was with the bat SARS-like coronavirus strain BatCov RaTG13, identity 96%."(11)

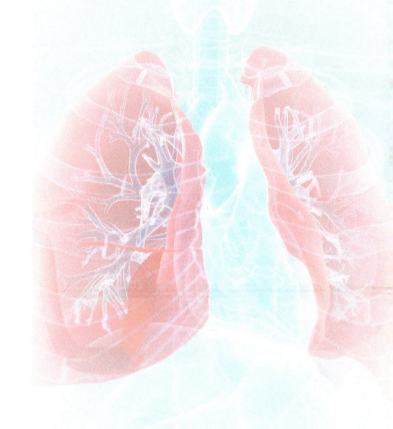

"Whole genome sequencing analysis of 104 strains of the COVID-19 virus isolated from patients in different localities with symptom onset between the end of December 2019 and mid-February 2020 showed 99.9% homology, without significant mutation" and are shown below.(11)

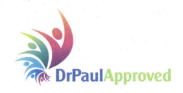

The illness caused by SARS-CoV-2 was initially called COVID-19 by the WHO, for "coronavirus disease 2019." On February 11, 2020, the Coronavirus Study Group of the International Committee on Taxonomy of Viruses announced the official designation for the novel virus would be severe acute respiratory syndrome coronavirus 2 (SARS-CoV-2).(12)

Severe acute respiratory syndrome (SARS) and Middle East respiratory syndrome (MERS) are the two coronavirus infections most like the SARS-CoV-2 that is the cause of the current pandemic. Over 8,000 individuals developed SARS, and almost 800 died (mortality rate of approximately 10%), before it was controlled in 2003. [28] MERS cases are still sporadic with about 2,465 laboratory- confirmed cases of MERS reported since 2012, and 850 deaths (mortality rate of 34.5%).

The SARS-CoV-2 is a group 2b beta-coronavirus that is 70% similar in genetic sequence to SARS-CoV and MERS-CoV. (13)

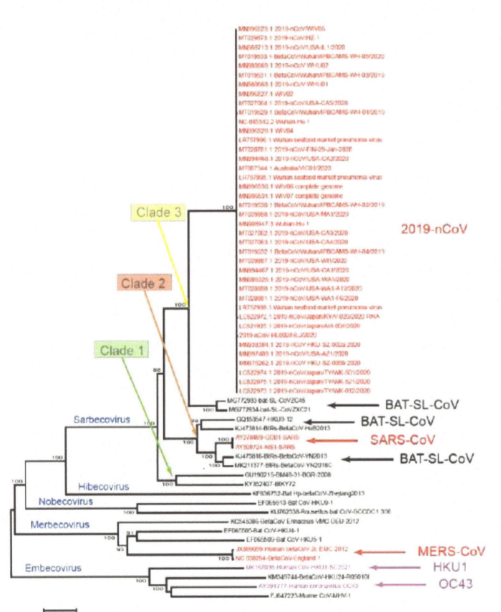

PHYLOGENETIC ANALYSIS OF THE COVID-19 VIRUS AND ITS CLOSELY RELATED REFERENCE GENOMES (12)

Note: COVID-19 virus is referred to as 2019-nCoV in the figure, the interim virus name WHO announced early in the outbreak.

The information in this book is educational and Informational only: IT IS NOT MEDICAL ADVICE. It is not intended to diagnose or treat. No pharmaceutical or dietary supplement has been proven in long-term placebo-controlled studies to treat or prevent COVID-19.

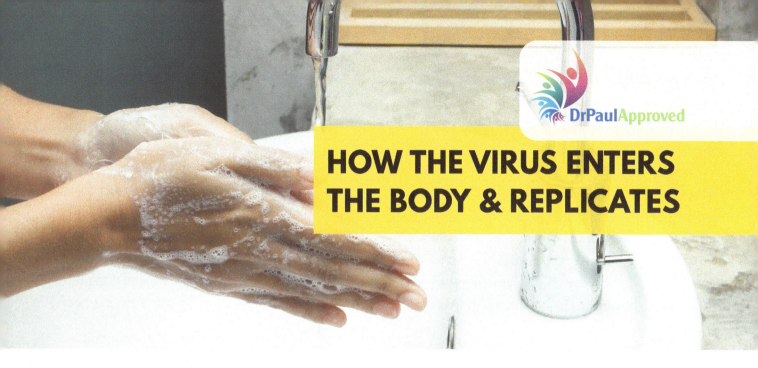

HOW THE VIRUS ENTERS THE BODY & REPLICATES

**COVID-19:
From your hands to your face.**

1. Keep your hands CLEAN at all times
2. Don't touch your face

COVID-19 is spread by direct contact when you touch someone who has the virus, or you touch a surface that was contaminated by the virus. Surfaces are most likely contaminated when a person with the virus touches objects that you then touch with your hands. When your hands reach your face, you have self-inoculated the virus to your body. Coughing and sneezing can send droplets into the air, hence the importance of covering your cough with your elbow if you might be sick or wearing a mask if you are sick. The earliest reports questioned whether it is possible to get the virus by breathing it in. The comprehensive WHO report states "airborne spread has not been reported for COVID-19 and it is not believed to be a major driver of transmission based on available evidence; however, it can be envisaged if certain aerosol-generating procedures are conducted in health care facilities."(11)

However, there is increasing evidence that transmission through the air is possible and even likely in certain situations. Medical procedures like intubation, and other hospital procedures on COVID-19 patients increase the likelihood of breathing in air containing the virus. The report of a choir practice in Washington on March 10, which likely transmitted the SARS-CoV-2 virus to approximately 40 of 60 choir members, highlights not only the airborne potential of transmission, but also the reality that people without symptoms can transmit this virus.(14) The study of seven clusters of COVID-19 infections in Singapore suggests that infected individuals are contagious for 1 - 3 days before they start to develop symptoms.(14) Since we know some people can have this virus and have no symptoms, clearly relying on identification and quarantine of the ill, by itself, will not contain this outbreak once it is well established in a community. This is why, during times of pandemic such as these, the avoidance of gatherings and keeping social distance is so important. It also may make sense to wear masks or at least cover our mouth and nose when out where close contact with others can occur.

The information in this book is educational and Informational only: IT IS NOT MEDICAL ADVICE. It is not intended to diagnose or treat. No pharmaceutical or dietary supplement has been proven in long-term placebo-controlled studies to treat or prevent COVID-19.

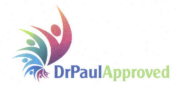

The virus has been identified in stool, and it is unclear at this time the extent to which fecal shedding is thought to be driving this pandemic. A number of studies suggest the possibility of fecal-oral transmission.(15)(16) The virus has been detected in stool for days and sometimes weeks after infection. In one study of 71 COVID-19 patients, the virus was found in the stool of 39 of the patients.(15) Furthermore, in 17 of the patients, the stool was positive for SARS-CoV-2 even after respiratory samples were negative for the virus. This is why good hand washing after using the bathroom or helping someone with toileting is vital.

The importance of this cannot be overstated. You can avoid this infection – even if you are a health care worker by never, ever, EVER, touching your face and washing your hands EVERY time you touch anything outside your home. Of course you'll need to think through how to avoid bringing this into your home.

If there is an elderly person, medically fragile person, or someone in your home who is immunocompromised or with major underlying health conditions, you simply cannot afford to take the risk of having visitors – PERIOD! Most of the secondary infections (78%-85%) are occurring in households with a household infection rate that appears to be in the 3% - 10% range.(11)

Tips for keeping COVID-19 out of your house

1. Leave your house only to exercise outdoors or get essentials.
2. Sanitize your house, including door knobs inside and out.
3. When in a store or touching anything, assume it has COVID-19 on it.
4. Either wear gloves or sanitize before and after touching anything.
5. If you wore gloves, don't take them into your car or home.
6. When bringing shipped items into the house, leave cardboard boxes outside.
7. Wash all produce and set to one side, then sanitize the side it was sitting on.
8. Sanitize all contents of purchases that are coming into your home.
9. If you can leave new purchases in the garage or shed for 2 days before bringing into the home.
10. Keep visitors out of your home. Anything they touch must be cleaned.
11. When out in public cover your face (mask if you have one or bandana).

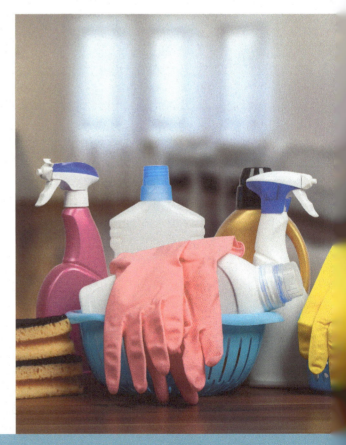

The information in this book is educational and Informational only: IT IS NOT MEDICAL ADVICE. It is not intended to diagnose or treat. No pharmaceutical or dietary supplement has been proven in long-term placebo-controlled studies to treat or prevent COVID-19.

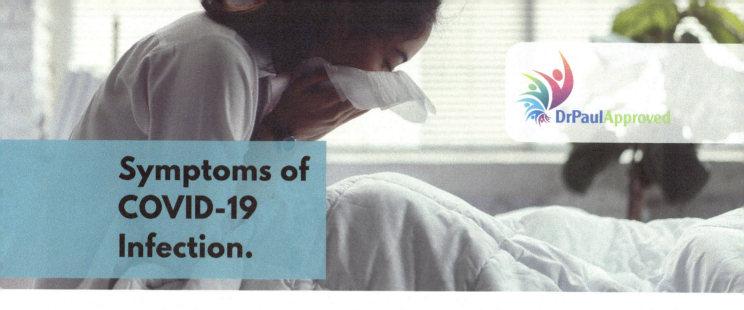

Symptoms of COVID-19 Infection.

Based on 55,924 laboratory confirmed cases, typical signs and symptoms include:

Symptoms of COVID-19

1. Fever (87.9%),
2. Dry cough (67.7%),
3. Fatigue (38.1%),
4. Sputum, wet cough (33.4%),
5. Shortness of breath (18.6%),
6. Sore throat (13.9%),
7. Headache (13.6%),
8. Myalgia -muscle aches or arthralgia - joint pain (14.8%),
9. Chills (11.4%),
10. Nausea or Vomiting (5.0%),
11. Nasal congestion (4.8%),
12. Diarrhea (3.7%),
13. hemoptysis – spitting up blood (0.9%),
14. Conjunctival congestion -red or swollen eyes (0.8%).

(Data based on 55,924 laboratory confirmed cases in China.(11)

Reports of loss of the sense of smell are surfacing. (17) Indeed I have a close friend whose daughter was in college overseas and returned with COVID-19 infection, and the only symptom was the loss of smell.

Most who get COVID-19 will recover. With an average time from infection to the start of symptoms (incubation) of 5 days and a range of up to 14 days, you would need to isolate yourself for two weeks if exposed to a known infection to be sure that you don't have the virus so you don't transmit it to others.

Most people who get infected with the virus causing COVID-19 will have mild symptoms like mild cough and fever and recover. About 13% end up with severe lung disease (defined as having shortness of breath or oxygen saturation ≤93%, or if you as an adult are breathing faster than 30 breaths a minute), and only 6.1% end up in critical condition (respiratory failure, septic shock, and/or multiple organ dysfunction/failure).(11)

The SARS- CoV-2 virus binds to cells of the lung, intestine, kidney and blood vessels through angiotensin-converting enzyme 2 (ACE2) receptors.(18) Conditions that make this receptor more abundant or active may put us at greater risk for a COVID-19 infection, since you are giving the virus more opportunity to bind and enter your body. These conditions include:

1. Type 1 or 2 diabetics, who are treated with ACE inhibitors and angiotensin II type-I receptor blockers (ARBs).(18)
2. High Blood Pressure (hypertension) patients treated with ACE inhibitors and ARBs.(19)

How the virus replicates

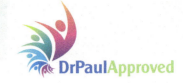

RNA viruses like SARS cannot survive without a host cell where they basically hijack your cells. The SARS-CoV-2 uses our cell's enzyme mTOR (mammalian target of rapamycin) to replicate. mTOR is basically what controls cell growth. After taking over the cell, SARS-CoV-2 can rapidly divide eventually filling up the cells until it bursts and releases a whole bunch more to infect the next cells nearby.

How SARS-CoV-2 causes ARDS (Adult Respiratory Distress Syndrome) – the main cause of death.

When our body is under attack and infected, we mount our defense with an inflammatory response. This brings added blood flow, beneficial nutrients and white blood cells to the site of injury to kill the infection, remove debris (dead cells) and generate new tissue. If, however, that inflammation is too extreme or goes on too long (chronic inflammation), this is where we get in trouble. In the case of SARS-CoV-2, in the lungs, the massive immune response starts to fill the lungs with fluid, and we can no longer oxygenate our blood. We are literally drowning in our own massive immune response. Most deaths from the COVID-19 infection are due to this process, which is called ARDS (Adult Respiratory Distress Syndrome).

The inflammatory process is sometimes called the inflammasome. The agents that get activated are called cytokines, with interleukins, like IL-1B, being specifically implicated as a cause of ARDS.[20] Studies are showing that SARS-CoV-2 is activating NOD, LLR and NLRP3 to release not only IL-1B but also IL-18 and that these are the main inflammation promoters that trigger ARDS.[21][22]

The initial reports out of Wuhan, China were that about ¾ of infections were men, usually older and 1/3 had underlying health conditions. They presented with fever (98%), cough (76%), and body aches or fatigue (44%) with headaches, sputum production and diarrhea less common. As they got worse more than half developed shortness of breath and 2/3 developed low levels of a white blood cell called lymphocytes (lymphopenia).[23][24]

All who had pneumonia had abnormal lung imaging findings, with acute respiratory distress syndrome (ARDS) developing in 29% of patients,[25] and ground-glass opacities a common finding on CT scans.[26]

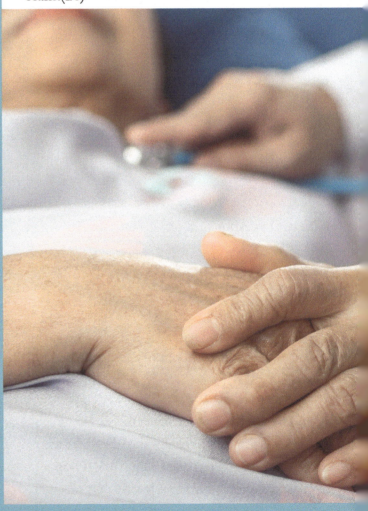

The information in this book is educational and Informational only: IT IS NOT MEDICAL ADVICE. It is not intended to diagnose or treat. No pharmaceutical or dietary supplement has been proven in long-term placebo-controlled studies to treat or prevent COVID-19.

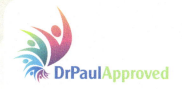

It is becoming clear that this virus is shared from person to person by respiratory droplets and hand-to-mouth exposures. If someone with this virus is coughing or sneezing, as with the common cold or flu, that will spread this virus, though SARS-CoV-2 is likely spread mostly by touching a contaminated surface rather than actually breathing in the virus from the air. Another interesting characteristic of the virus is that very few young children seem to get sick and they seem to have mild illness.(27)

What is clearly making it difficult to control the spread of COVID-19 is that people without any symptoms can carry the virus and infect others. This is actually a reason the world-wide approach of isolation, while helpful at reducing the speed of transmission, will likely fail to stop the spread of this virus. A recent study found increases in viral loads at the time that the patients became symptomatic, with one patient who never developed symptoms shedding the virus beginning at day 7 after a presumed infection.(28) It seems the epidemic is doubling about every 3 - 7 days, and the base reproductive number was 2.2, meaning every patient infects an average of 2.2 others.(29)

As a busy pediatrician, I have seen hundreds of patients this past winter with flu-like symptoms that included high fevers and cough, sometimes with headaches and body aches. In my office, if a child is particularly sick looking, we will do a rapid flu (influenza A and B) and RSV (Respiratory Syncytial Virus), test and sometimes a comprehensive respiratory panel along with a CBC (complete blood count). In November and December, we were identifying lots of influenza A and in January RSV and influenza B.

We also, however, were having an unusual number of children with low white counts and relative lymphopenia (low number of the white blood cells known as lymphocytes) and negative respiratory panels, meaning they did not have influenza A, B RSV or anything else for that matter. COVID-19 was not yet on our radar!

To make a COVID-19 diagnosis we need to get a positive test. This means that we are likely under-diagnosing these infections. In my State or Oregon, in late March 2020, only 5% of all tests for COVID-19 have been positive and this at a time when testing is only being offered to the very ill. I have sent in a few tests and so far, all have returned negative. At this time in the USA, when other tests like those for the flu are negative, we are only testing the very ill or the moderately ill, as well as people who have come in close contact with positive cases. If laboratory testing confirms an alternate pathogen, SARS-CoV-2 can be considered excluded, although this could change in the future as it is certainly possible to have more than one infection at the same time.(30)

The CDC developed a real-time reverse transcription-polymerase chain reaction (rRT-PCR) assay that can be used to diagnose the virus in respiratory and serum samples.(31)

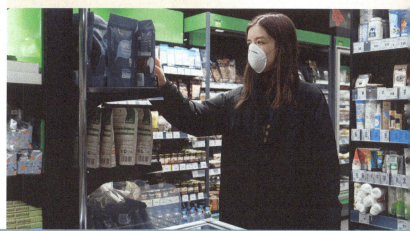

The information in this book is educational and Informational only: IT IS NOT MEDICAL ADVICE. It is not intended to diagnose or treat. No pharmaceutical or dietary supplement has been proven in long-term placebo-controlled studies to treat or prevent COVID-19.

RNA viruses like SARS cannot survive without a host cell where they basically hijack your cells. The SARS-CoV-2 uses our cell's enzyme mTOR (mammalian target of rapamycin) to replicate. mTOR is basically what controls cell growth. After taking over the cell, SARS-CoV-2 can rapidly divide eventually filling up the cells until it bursts and releases a whole bunch more to infect the next cells nearby.

How SARS-CoV-2 causes ARDS (Adult Respiratory Distress Syndrome) – the main cause of death.

When our body is under attack and infected, we mount our defense with an inflammatory response. This brings added blood flow, beneficial nutrients and white blood cells to the site of injury to kill the infection, remove debris (dead cells) and generate new tissue. If, however, that inflammation is too extreme or goes on too long (chronic inflammation), this is where we get in trouble. In the case of SARS-CoV-2, in the lungs, the massive immune response starts to fill the lungs with fluid, and we can no longer oxygenate our blood. We are literally drowning in our own massive immune response. Most deaths from the COVID-19 infection are due to this process, which is called ARDS (Adult Respiratory Distress Syndrome).

The inflammatory process is sometimes called the inflammasome. The agents that get activated are called cytokines, with interleukins, like IL-1B, being specifically implicated as a cause of ARDS.(20) Studies are showing that SARS-CoV-2 is activating NOD, LLR and NLRP3 to release not only IL-1B but also IL-18 and that these are the main inflammation promoters that trigger ARDS.(21)(22)

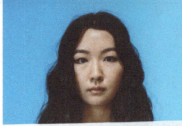
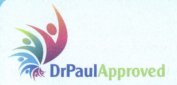

The China Experience

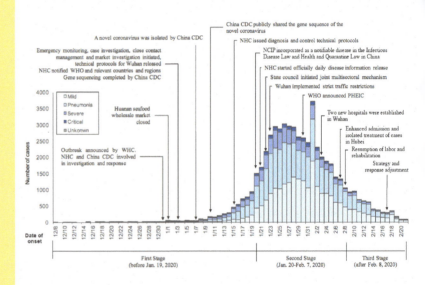

Source: World Health Organization(12)

The initial reports out of Wuhan, China were that about ¾ of infections were men, usually older and 1/3 had underlying health conditions. They presented with fever (98%), cough (76%), and body aches or fatigue (44%) with headaches, sputum production and diarrhea less common. As they got worse more than half developed shortness of breath and 2/3 developed low levels of a white blood cell called lymphocytes (lymphopenia).(23)(24)

All who had pneumonia had abnormal lung imaging findings, with acute respiratory distress syndrome (ARDS) developing in 29% of patients,(25) and ground-glass opacities a common finding on CT scans.(26)

The information in this book is educational and Informational only: IT IS NOT MEDICAL ADVICE. It is not intended to diagnose or treat. No pharmaceutical or dietary supplement has been proven in long-term placebo-controlled studies to treat or prevent COVID-19.

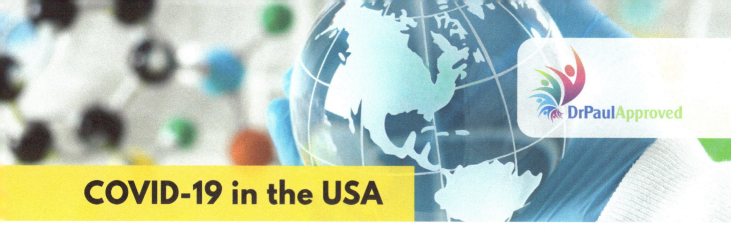

COVID-19 in the USA

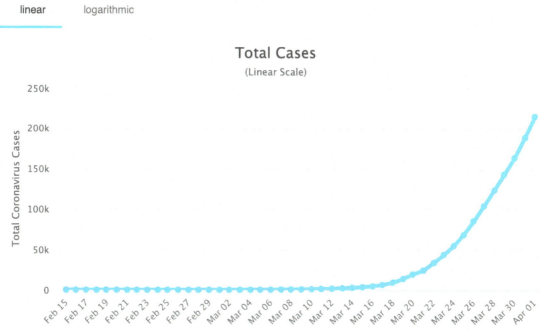

This image is from April 2, 2020.
Source: https://www.worldometers.info/coronavirus/

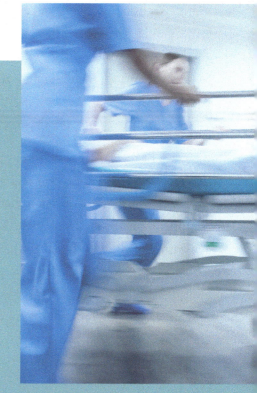

This does not look like the flattening of the curve that all the Government and health officials have been calling for. In theory, flattening the curve seems to be essential to avoid overwhelming the medical system, hospitals and our supply of ventilators. The main reason for this may be that by the time new cases are identified in any location there are already many more people infected who don't realize they are.

Each day since our first reported case in Everett, Washington on January 5, 2020 all you have to do is turn on the news to see that across the country we are seeing a massive rise in numbers identified and deaths. The statistic missing, is the numbers tested, but it is becoming painfully clear, that our testing capabilities have blinded us to the realities of how widespread COVID-19 is in the USA. Unless you live in a very small and isolated place where outsiders don't visit, chances are the epidemic is already growing in your community.

The information in this book is educational and Informational only: IT IS NOT MEDICAL ADVICE. It is not intended to diagnose or treat. No pharmaceutical or dietary supplement has been proven in long-term placebo-controlled studies to treat or prevent COVID-19.

FLATTENING THE CURVE

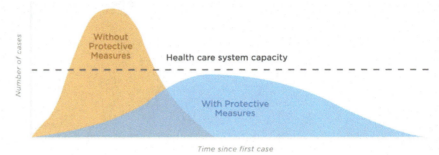

Source: CDC, Drew Harris   Credit: Connie Hanzhang Jin/NPR

There is a very steep curve portrayed here for "without protective measures." This seems to match the experience in most countries, including the USA, at this time. We all must do what we can to prepare for things to get worse while doing everything possible to boost our own immune systems so that we can withstand the virus when we get exposed. Count on getting exposed despite your best efforts and count on not getting that ill because you will be making vital lifestyle changes and supporting your immune system, which may minimize the viral impact on your body and enable you to beat this.

New cases seem to be doubling about every 2 to 3 days. While part of this is due to the expanded testing that is being done, there is no question that COVID-19 is a formidable foe. Continue to do all you can to honor social distancing and avoid indoor crowds and gatherings. The massive school and business closings will certainly help to slow the spread. Avoiding indoor close contact with groups of people is surely one of the most important things we can do.

The lack of testing frankly has resulted in the need for all of us, citizens and medical professionals, to make decisions based on very incomplete data. If we knew that only 1 in a million children under the age of 10 or 15 or 18 would die and that young adults, and their parents would also fare well as long as they had no underlying medical conditions, we could consider quarantine for the elderly and those at high risk.

Since we have no idea what percentage of the population exposed gets little to no symptoms, what percentage gets a mild flu-like illness and what percentage gets severely ill and dies, we are left with this need to shut down our entire way of life.

Global mortality is around 3.7% of those tested, but these rates are massively inflated because for most countries and for the USA we simply don't have enough tests. Only the very ill get tested and their close contacts so of course mortality seems high. Countries with good access to testing and whose governments have taken swift action to contain the virus have much lower mortality rates. If we begin massive testing that includes those only minimally ill or perhaps even those who are not ill, then we will see mortality rates plummet.

Images out of Italy of hospitals overflowing with people lined up on ventilators and caskets being trucked out on a massive scale make it crystal clear – this is nothing like anything any of us have seen in our lifetimes. We are starting to see the same happen in the USA, and hot spots around the world. Be aware, however, that images on the television can sometimes be manipulated. We need to verify everything as time goes on to be sure that we really have the right data, an accurate picture of the real events on the ground so we don't give up our civil liberties out of drummed up fear. In Portland, Oregon where we are preparing for the massive wave of severe cases, hospitals are still like ghost towns, the tents outside the ER's empty. If we have flattened the curve in a massive way –wonderful! Where else has this happened?

I want you to be empowered to do anything and everything, so you and your loved ones survive this. We will look back with gratitude for having survived this and with great sorrow for all those lost. I hope we don't throw out our freedom and way of life in the process. There will be a before 2020 and an after 2020 sense of things. If we are wise and vigilant to the actual reasons behind this devastating pandemic, we can avoid mistakes of the past and prepare our immune systems for any future such threats.

TREATMENT OPTIONS

Once you are hospitalized, you are put in total isolation, and no family or visitors are generally allowed. Your options at this point tend to be limited to those standard treatments the establishment is aware of. As pneumonia gets worse, your lungs fill with fluid and for some the only way to survive is intubation and being on a ventilator.

Reports are now coming of success for those who are intubated or have organ failure, with the use of convalescent plasma. This basically takes the plasma (the clear part of our blood that has all the antibodies etc.) from a person who has recovered and gives this intravenously (in your vein) to the patient. While only 5 patients are reported in this study, they all survived.(33)

On March 22, The New York Times reported a potential 69 existing drugs or compounds that might be effective in treating the coronavirus. (34) We are hearing reports of benefits from chloroquine and also from chloroquine given with azithromycin.(35) The articles of various antivirals and other pharmaceuticals that may help will be pouring out faster than anyone can keep up with, so our knowledge will explode by the day.

The key for most who read this book is doing everything you can BEFORE you need hospitalization. It will be a rare intensive care doctor who would be open to the treatments below, once you are hospitalized and especially if you are intubated. Most hospitals have a policy that you cannot bring into the hospital "outside medications" and vitamins and supplements apparently are included in that designation.

TREATMENT GOALS:

1. Prevent SARS-CoV-2 from entering the body
2. Slow its replication and ability to damage our cells
3. Kill the virus
4. Recover from infection.

The hippocratic oath we physicians are supposed to abide by is to First Do No Harm.

I'd like to propose that we expand this concept so that each and every physician embraces approaches that they may not be familiar with or even comfortable with, as long as they pose little threat of harm and may in fact be very beneficial to the patient. If you deny your patient a treatment that might benefit them due to your lack of humility or knowledge or understanding – are you really "doing no harm?" We allow compassionate use for much more dangerous unproven and experimental cancer drugs when they might help.

The media, our public health officials and mainstream medicine colleagues need to embrace anything and everything that might help you avoid a serious infection or recover from a COVID-19 infection, especially if it has a great safety profile.

Here's more information on the science supporting the use of supplements that may support a healthy immune system both in people who want to reduce their risk of COVID-19 and people who have already contracted the virus.

The information in this book is educational and Informational only: IT IS NOT MEDICAL ADVICE. It is not intended to diagnose or treat. No pharmaceutical or dietary supplement has been proven in long-term placebo-controlled studies to treat or prevent COVID-19.

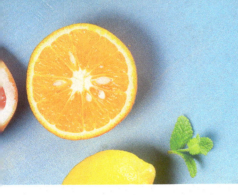
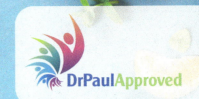

VITAMIN C

The SARS-CoV-2 virus has a unique ability to destroy or consume our lymphocytes. Patients in Wuhan who were in critical condition would survive if in the third week of infection they could still produce lymphocytes, and those who could not, usually died.(36) Our T-lymphocytes are vital in fighting viral infections and vitamin C is important for T-lymphocyte production in our body.(37)(38) The lymphocytes called natural killer (NK) cells are particularly important to fight off a viral infection. Vitamin C boosts NK cell production and function.(39)

On March 3, 2020, government officials in Shanghai, China announced the recommendation that COVID-19 should be treated with high amounts of intravenous vitamin C.(40) The intravenous doses- range from 50 to 200 milligrams per kilogram of body weight per day, or 4,000 to 16,000 mg for an adult.

Dr. Yanagisawa, MD, PhD, president of the Tokyo-based Japanese College of Intravenous Therapy, stated that vitamin C's effect is at least ten times more powerful by IV than if taken orally. He went on to say that "Intravenous vitamin C is a safe, effective, and broad-spectrum antiviral."

Xi'an Jiaotong University Second Hospital made the following official statement: "On the afternoon of February 20, 2020, another 4 patients with severe new coronaviral pneumonia recovered from the C10 West Ward of Tongji Hospital. In the past 8 patients have been discharged from hospital... [H]igh-dose vitamin C achieved good results in clinical applications. We believe that for patients with severe neonatal pneumonia and critically ill patients, vitamin C treatment should be initiated as soon as possible after admission...[E]arly application of large doses of vitamin C can have a strong antioxidant effect, reduce inflammatory responses, and improve endothelial function... Numerous studies have shown that the dose of vitamin C has a lot to do with the effect of treatment... [H]gh-dose vitamin C can not only improve antiviral levels, but more importantly, can prevent and treat acute lung injury (ALI) and acute respiratory distress (ARDS)."(41)

The use of vitamin C for viral infections is well established in the literature.(42)(43)(44)(45)(46) The literature on vitamin C benefits includes evidence that even small amounts of vitamin C can keep severely ill patients from dying.(47) There was reduced mortality in Infants with viral pneumonia treated with vitamin C.(48)

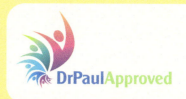

While a meta-analysis showed an overall reduction of 8% for duration of ICU stays for those given vitamin C one study showed that high vitamin C given intravenously shortened intensive care unit stay by 44%.(49) A mere 200 mg of vitamin C reduced the duration of severe pneumonia in children, and oxygen saturation improved in less than one day.(50)

Humans have basically lost their ability to make their own vitamin C. This is in contrast to most other animals which makes us uniquely vulnerable to depletion of this essential nutrient. The genetic defect whereby we lost the ability to synthesize ascorbate is caused by a mutated defective gene for the liver enzyme, L-gulonolactone oxidase.(51)

The higher mammals (except for the higher primates and humans) developed a feedback mechanism which increases ascorbate synthesis under the influence of external and internal stresses.(52)(53) Our inability to produce more vitamin C during stress and infection is the basis for our need for more during these times. The amount needed to maintain health during normal times where stress is low and you do not have an infection is probably quite low, in the range of 250 mg to 4 grams a day for an adult. Note the RDA (Recommended Daily Allowance) for vitamin C, which is that amount needed to prevent scurvy, is 15 – 50 mg for infants and children and 75 – 120 mg for those over age 13.(54)

As we think about viral infections and stress as perhaps the two most vitamin C depleting events for our bodies, this current COVID-19 pandemic is perhaps creating the greatest need for more vitamin C in the past century!

Our bodies, when well-nourished, only store about 5 grams (5,000 mg) of vitamin C.(55) With the major source of vitamin C being fresh fruits and vegetables, most of us are in a state of vitamin C deficiency, and at risk for many problems related to failure of metabolic processes dependent upon vitamin C. We might think of this as a chronic scurvy. Since vitamin C is vital for our immune system, connective tissue, heart and blood vessel health, and our ability to handle stress, this may be the key to surviving times of serious stress or infection.

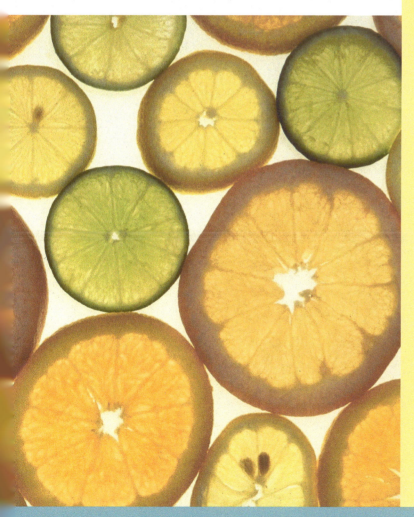

The information in this book is educational and Informational only: IT IS NOT MEDICAL ADVICE. It is not intended to diagnose or treat. No pharmaceutical or dietary supplement has been proven in long-term placebo-controlled studies to treat or prevent COVID-19.

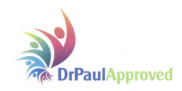

One of the important ways vitamin C helps us get rid of COVID-19 is that vitamin C supports our glutathione, keeping it in the active form of reduced glutathione. As glutathione does its job, it is oxidized, and without vitamin C to help it back to the active reduced form it is useless. In the active form, glutathione supports our white blood cells (neutrophils) in the process called phagocytosis, where they literally gobble up the virus to destroy it. Without enough glutathione those same neutrophils can switch from the beneficial phagocytosis to degranulation that is basically blowing up and destroying the cell and the tissue around the cell. In severe COVID-19 infections, this is likely a big part of the inflammatory storm that results in the lung damage and need for intubation and even death.

Acetaminophen (Tylenol®) blocks the production of glutathione.(56) Taking acetaminophen is probably the absolute last thing you should do when fighting a serious COVID-19 infection, and yet the shelves in the stores are empty after some TV report that ibuprofen was bad for COVID-19 (which it might be) and people were advised to stock up on Tylenol®.

How Much Vitamin C Can You Take Orally?

It turns out most of us can tolerate between 4 and 15 grams (4,000 - 15,000 mg) of vitamin C daily before we develop diarrhea.

```
TABLE I - USUAL BOWEL TOLERANCE DOSES

                        GRAMS ASCORBIC ACID   NUMBER OF DOSE
CONDITION                 PER 24 HOURS         PER 24 HOURS
  normal                     4  -   15            4  -   6
  mild cold                 30  -   60            6  -  10
  severe cold               60  -  100+           8  -  15
  influenza                100  -  150            8  -  20
  ECHO, coxsackievirus     100  -  150            8  -  20
  mononucleosis            150  -  200+          12  -  25
  viral pneumonia          100  -  200+          12  -  25
  hay fever, asthma         15  -   50            4  -   8
  environmental and
    food allergy           0.5  -   50            4  -   8
  burn, injury, surgery     25  -  150+           6  -  20
  anxiety, exercise and
    other mild stresses     15  -   25            4  -   6
  cancer                    15  -  100            4  -  15
  ankylosing spondylitis    15  -  100            4  -  15
  Reiter's syndrome         15  -   60            4  -  10
  acute anterior uveitis    30  -  100            4  -  15
  rheumatoid arthritis      15  -  100            4  -  15
  bacterial infections      30  -  200+          10  -  25
  infectious hepatitis      30  -  100            6  -  15
  candidiasis               15  -  200+           6  -  25
```

Source: Robert F. Cathcart, III, M.D. Vitamin C, Titrating to Bowel Tolerance, Anascorbemia, and Acute Induced Scurvy. Medical Hypotheses, 7:1359-1376, 1981.

Doctors and anyone for that matter, using vitamin C at high doses, have learned that your tolerance for vitamin C can change. We actually tolerate much higher doses when we are ill as the table above demonstrates.

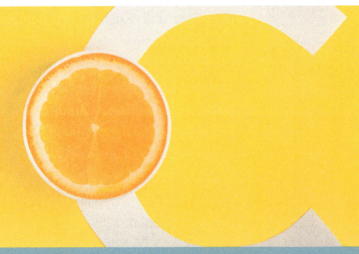

Bowel Tolerance

We have learned that the amount of ascorbic acid (vitamin C) we can take orally without causing diarrhea when ill can be ten times the amount we would tolerate if well. Maximum benefit from oral vitamin C seems to be at the highest dose you can tolerate, just short of the dose that causes you diarrhea. This means each person should alter their dose and frequency to match their circumstance. From Part 1, you can see that I was recommending very high doses for those potentially infected with COVID-19. How often you should take your vitamin C orally could be as infrequent as twice a day when you are well to every 10 - 15 minutes if you are close to hospitalization due to severe COVID-19 infection, and getting air hungry, or experiencing extreme fevers and fatigue.

Basically, adjust your dose between the amount that makes you feel better and the amount that starts to cause diarrhea.

A Note to the Skeptics

You will undoubtedly encounter skeptics of this vitamin C role in our fight against COVID-19. You can find articles that show vitamin C makes no difference in protecting you from infections. Common to all such studies is the use of doses that are too small to make a difference. Imagine studying the effect of morphine on pain but using a dose that was 1/10 the known effective dose, or 1/10 acetaminophen or 1/10 ibuprofen. The results would be unanimous: these medications are worthless for pain management. It is no different here for vitamin C. The only difference perhaps is that relatively low doses of vitamin C might still have benefit, and if very ill, very high doses may be needed.

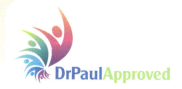

What other doctors have said about high-dose vitamin C

Dr. Linus Pauling, Nobel prize winner and vitamin C expert, published Vitamin C and the Common Cold, a book that revolutionized the way the world viewed vitamin C and infectious disease.(57)

Dr. Andrew W. Saul, an international expert on vitamin therapy, says, "The coronavirus can be dramatically slowed or stopped completely with the immediate widespread use of high doses of vitamin C. Bowel tolerance levels of C taken in divided doses throughout the day, is a clinically proven antiviral, without equal."

Dr. Thomas Levy, M.D., J.D., board-certified cardiologist recommends inclusion of liposomal form of C in fighting viral and other diseases, in his book "Curing the Incurable Vitamin C, Infectious Diseases, and Toxins".

From clinical trials in China, Dr. Cheng, MD, PhD and his colleagues: "Increased oxidative stress, an underlying 'cytokine storm,' leads to ARDS which is the key pathology of high mortality of these pandemic viral infections. Intravenous vitamin C effectively counters oxidative stress." Registered clinical trials on Vitamin C and COVID-19.(58)

For a recent webinar on the use of vitamin C by Paul Anderson a respected expert of IV vitamin C, International Society for Orthomolecular Medicine website: https://isom.ca/vitamin-c-coronavirus/

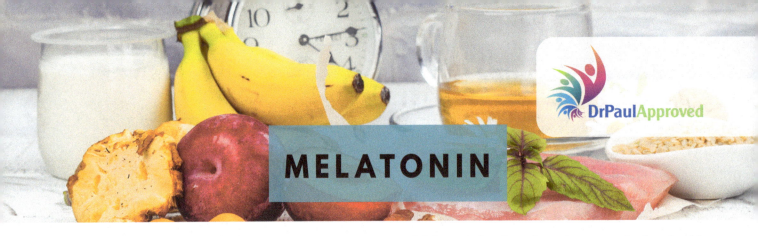

MELATONIN

While melatonin reduces inflammation, it is not specifically antiviral. However, the inflammation that melatonin can reduce is exactly the process that is contributing to respiratory failure and other systemic effects of COVID-19 that likely ends up killing patients.

There is evidence that melatonin can stop apoptosis, the process in which infected cells with a virus actually kill themselves trying to stop the spread of the disease.(59) Although apoptosis is helpful in some diseases, in the end stages of COVID-19 infection, when patients are needing a ventilator, slowing down the inflammation and apoptosis is undoubtedly going to help.

Below is a table showing the age-associated production of melatonin.(60)

Melatonin has long been known to be involved in promoting sleep but it appears to also target the NLRP inflammasomes directly. Melatonin has been shown to limit damage in animal models of sepsis by this mechanism.(61)(62)(63) Melatonin helps maintain normal lung mitochondrial function protecting the lungs of the elderly from the normal decline that occurs with aging.(64) In mice, studies have shown that supplemental melatonin reduces damage from acute lung injury, ARDS and mechanical ventilation.(65)

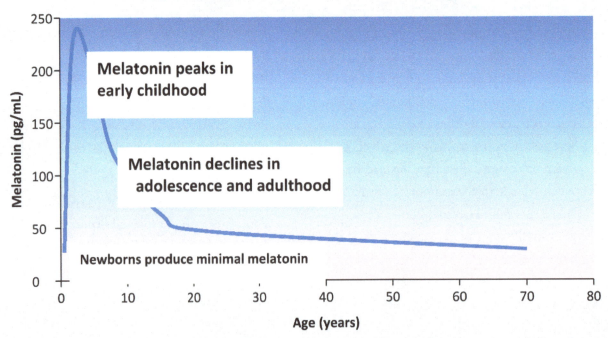

Melatonin Production With Age.

The information in this book is educational and Informational only: IT IS NOT MEDICAL ADVICE. It is not intended to diagnose or treat. No pharmaceutical or dietary supplement has been proven in long-term placebo-controlled studies to treat or prevent COVID-19.

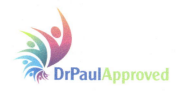

The peer reviewed article "COVID-19: Melatonin as a potential adjuvant treatment" outlines the various mechanisms by which melatonin may be helpful in the body's immune response against COVID-19.(66)

The authors wrote, "We postulated that lungs infected by SARS-CoV-2, and a suppressed immune response, elevated inflammation and excessive oxidation stress proceed unabated, this results in the activation of the cytokine storm.

ALI/ARDS may ensue, accompanied by a series of complications, the outcomes of which vary according to the severity of the disease. Melatonin may play a role of adjuvant medication in the regulation of the immune system, inflammation and oxidative stress, and provide support for patients with ALI/ARDS and related complications."(66)

Numerous studies are now published showing the lung protective benefits of melatonin during serious viral infections.(67)(68)(69)(70)(71)(72)

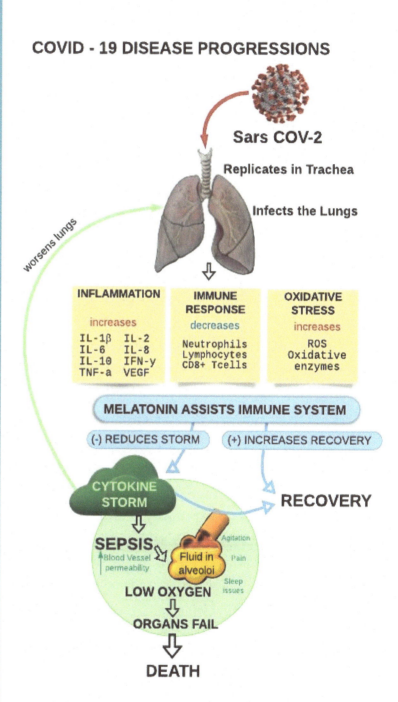

Source: https://www.sciencedirect.com/science/article/pii/S0024320520303313

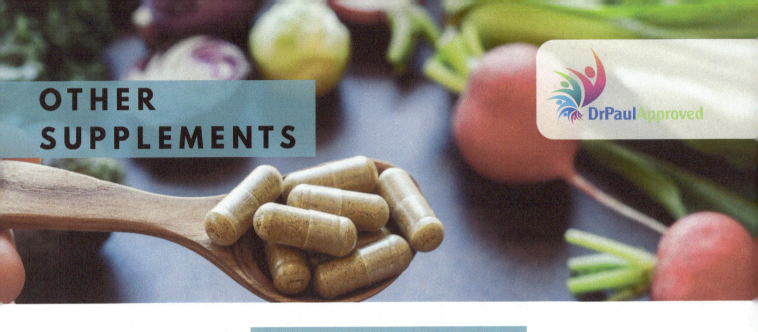

OTHER SUPPLEMENTS

VITAMIN D

Vitamin D is my "do not leave home without it" supplement. Virtually everyone in the world is deficient and this "vitamin," which is actually a hormone involved in many important pathways, including the vitality of our immune system. I highly recommend you supplement with Vitamin D3. I use a D3 supplement that has K2. Let me explain.

Simply put, vitamin D among its many roles, helps us absorb calcium from the food we eat. One theory as to why vitamin D may be causing adverse outcomes in some people (such as worse coronary artery related issues) is that without adequate K2 to help usher that calcium you're absorbing into the bones where it belongs, the calcium may be deposited in other areas of the body – like your blood vessels – where it can cause damage. Our bones act like the bank where extra calcium is stored. Classic vitamin D deficiency in children results in rickets, where bones with inadequate calcium are soft and kids can end up with bowed legs. Older adults often have osteopenia (bones that are poorly mineralized and more vulnerable to breaking).

Since the COVID-19 viral infection is so new there are no studies on vitamin D use with COVID-19.

We can, however, take note of the studies where vitamin D has made a difference in the ability to fight other infections like influenza (the flu).

Vitamin D affects our immune system in many specific ways. Down regulation of the cytokine storm discussed earlier is one important reason you want to have optimal vitamin D levels. Vitamin D inhibits Th1 and Th0 cells by inhibiting IL-2, IFNγ, and TNFα and promotes the production of Treg cells by facilitating production of IL-10. Vitamin D also promotes a Th2-mediated immune response by promoting IL-4, IL-5, and IL-10, and inhibits a Th17-mediated immune response by inhibiting IL-6 and IL-23. Vitamin D inhibits the production of B-cells their differentiation into plasma cells, and the production of antibodies by B-cells. In addition this immune balancing role vitamin D promotes antiviral and immunomodulatory interferon signaling.(73)

The information in this book is educational and Informational only: IT IS NOT MEDICAL ADVICE. It is not intended to diagnose or treat. No pharmaceutical or dietary supplement has been proven in long-term placebo-controlled studies to treat or prevent COVID-19.

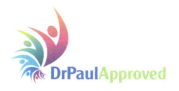

Vitamin D is the one vitamin that we generally cannot get enough of from a typical diet. We make most of our vitamin D when sunlight hits our skin. The fact that we are indoors most of the time and wear clothes and sunscreen when outdoors limits the amount of vitamin D we will make naturally. Vitamin D levels are lower in the winter months and the further away from the equator you are. There is also a direct correlation between low levels of vitamin D and increased incidence of influenza infections along with a reduction of influenza rates when you supplement with vitamin D.(74)(75) A similar association between low vitamin D levels and upper respiratory tract infections has been found.(76)

In a meta-analysis and systematic review of 25 studies with over 10,000 participants showed very significant benefits from supplementing with Vitamin D in the prevention of influenza.(77) The review authors concluded, "Vitamin D supplementation was safe and it protected against acute respiratory tract infection overall. Patients who were very vitamin D deficient and those not receiving bolus doses experienced the most benefit." This benefit was also found to be true for children.(78)

Since we know that individuals with underlying chronic conditions seem to be a higher risk for COVID-19 infections, it is reassuring to note that vitamin D supplementation seemed to help reduce influenza infections in those with inflammatory bowel disease.(79) In a recent study in children in Vietnam, researchers found vitamin D supplementation reduced non-influenza infections in children.(80) Infants seem to particularly benefit from vitamin D supplementation. According to a recent study, "High-dose vitamin D (1,200 IU) is suitable for the prevention of seasonal influenza as evidenced by rapid relief from symptoms, rapid decrease in viral loads, and disease recovery. In addition, high-dose vitamin D is probably safe for infants."(81)

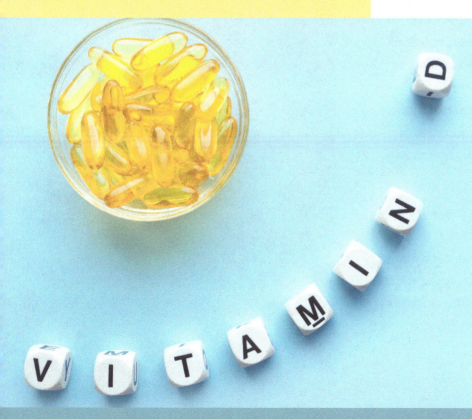

The information in this book is educational and Informational only: IT IS NOT MEDICAL ADVICE. It is not intended to diagnose or treat. No pharmaceutical or dietary supplement has been proven in long-term placebo-controlled studies to treat or prevent COVID-19.

So How Much Vitamin D Should You Take?

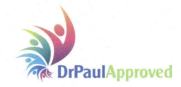

If you know you are deficient or if you have very little contact with sunlight on your skin or live far from the equator and you have not been supplementing with vitamin D3, I can assure you that you are deficient. I have tested thousands of children and young adults in my career and only those on high-dose supplementation (generally 5,000 IU a day for teens and adults, 2,000 IU for children and 1,000 IU for infants) have optimal levels, while most who are not supplementing vitamin D are significantly deficient. The experience of Canadian physician Gerry Schwalfenberg mirrors my own.

Dr. Schwalfenberg wrote, "A colleague of mine and I have introduced vitamin D at doses that have achieved greater than 100 nmol/L in most of our patients for the past number of years, and we now see very few patients in our clinics with the flu or influenza-like illness. In those patients who do have influenza, we have treated them with the vitamin D hammer, as coined by my colleague. This is a 1-time 50,000 IU dose of vitamin D3 or 10,000 IU 3 times daily for 2 to 3 days. The results are dramatic, with complete resolution of symptoms in 48 to 72 hours. One-time doses of vitamin D at this level have been used safely and have never been shown to be toxic."(82)

I have not had a single COVID-19 patient, nor have any of my staff had COVID-19 (at least that we know of). It is possible we are having mild symptoms and developing immunity. Most of my 15,000 patients and 35 staff know to take adequate vitamin D. Association does not prove anything. I merely share this as an observation.

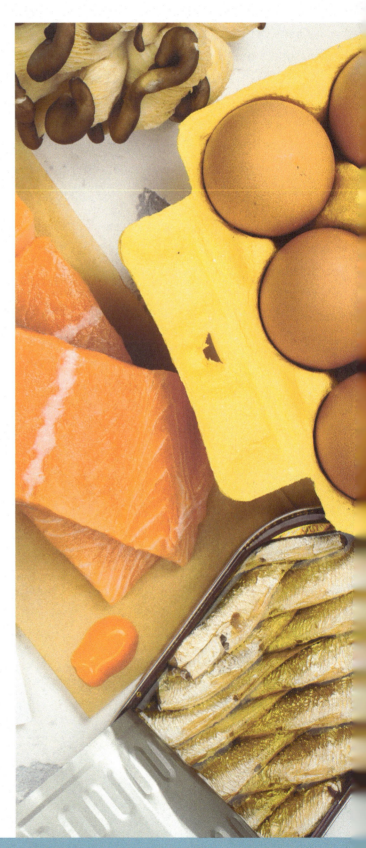

50

The information in this book is educational and Informational only: IT IS NOT MEDICAL ADVICE. It is not intended to diagnose or treat. No pharmaceutical or dietary supplement has been proven in long-term placebo-controlled studies to treat or prevent COVID-19.

MAGNESIUM SUPPLEMENTATION

When we supplement with high dose vitamin D, this can lower our magnesium levels. One challenge in the assessment of magnesium status is that the serum level in a blood test is a poor measure of magnesium in the body.(83) Magnesium is a cofactor in the production of ATP (adenosine triphosphate), the molecule that transfers energy, in the mitochondria. Since each human cell contains 1,000-2,000 mitochondria, magnesium this is a vital nutrient for normal function of our cells.(84)(85) Magnesium is needed for 600-800 enzyme processes.(86)(87)

If you are supplementing with high-dose vitamin D or calcium, it is important to know that magnesium is important for properly functioning muscles, allowing calcium to cause muscle contraction and then pushing calcium out of the muscle cells to allow the relaxation phase.(88) I recommend magnesium any time you supplement with calcium or if there are any muscle cramps. It is generally calming, so may be a worthy addition during times of stress as well. Make sure that your multivitamin has magnesium or that you are supplementing with this important mineral.

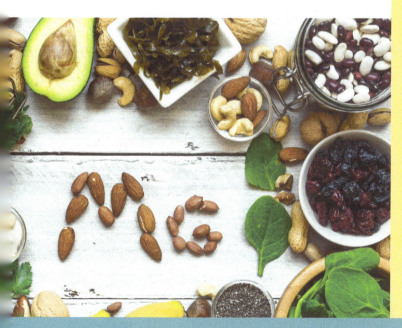

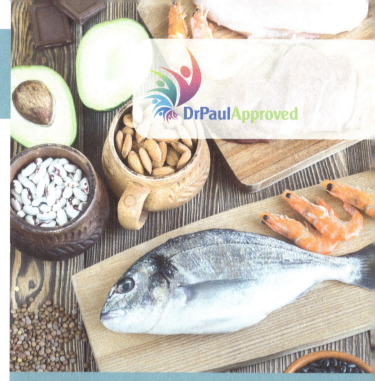

ZINC SUPPLEMENTATION

Zinc is intimately connected with immune function. Zinc deficiency rapidly diminishes antibody and cell-mediated responses, which are so vital in our battle against infections. Since we have learned that COVID-19 infections specifically reduce lymphocytes which is also a hallmark of zinc deficiency, replacing zinc is of vital importance when battling COVID-19 infections.(89) One of the mechanisms by which zinc helps the immune system is through the inhibition of NF-kB.(90)

Zinc is important for normal function of neutrophils and natural killer cells. It is also important for immune activation, Th1 cytokine production, and B lymphocyte antibody production. The macrophage is vital in our battle against infections and is adversely affected by zinc deficiency, which can dysregulate intracellular killing, cytokine production, and phagocytosis.(91)

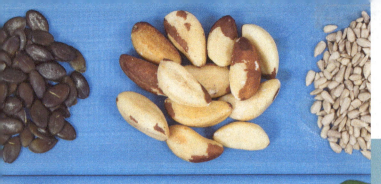
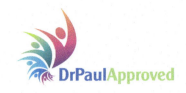
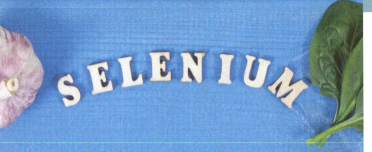

SELENIUM SUPPLEMENTATION - THE JURY IS STILL OUT

Selenium (Se) acts as a nutritional antioxidant through its incorporation into selenoproteins which regulate reactive oxygen species (ROS) and redox status, thus influencing inflammation and immune responses.(92)

Selenium can affect the function of cells of both adaptive and innate immunity. High dose selenium promotes proliferation and favors differentiation of naive CD4-positive T lymphocytes toward T helper 1 cells, thus supporting the acute cellular immune response. Excessive activation of the immune system can result in tissue damage which can be counteracted through directing macrophages toward the M2 phenotype.(93) While I usually support selenium supplementation when wanting to boost the immune system or support detox pathways, the jury is still out whether or not this is a good nutrient to supplement when faced with a COVID-19 infection.

THE ROLE OF CBD

I've been following the scientific explosion of information about cannabidiol (CBD). Recently the FDA (U.S. Food and Drug Administration) approved Epidiolex® (cannabidiol) oral solution for the treatment of seizures associated with two rare and severe forms of epilepsy, Lennox-Gastaut syndrome and Dravet syndrome, in patients two years of age and older.(94) This has opened the door for physicians to consider off label uses for conditions that seem to benefit from taking CBD.

Given the massive threat that the COVID-19 pandemic presents to the world, CBD may be worth considering. You will want to find a very pure source with minimal to no THC. I'm exploring a new product of very pure CBD made from the terpenes in orange peels and hope to have access to that product to share with you very soon.

The health of our immune systems has remained the top concern for my patients and everyone around the world. Consequently, discussing whether CBD oil can support immune health is a timely topic of conversation. CBD may be an important part of a complete immune support regimen, alongside other recommendations in this book and getting enough sleep, moderate exercise and avoiding processed, sugary foods.

CBD is a plant-based cannabinoid, a compound that works on a health-promoting system of your body known as the endocannabinoid system. Typically, CBD is extracted hemp. Hemp-derived CBD oils often have at least a small amount of THC, the compound in marijuana that makes you high, so be careful if using these products in children.

An analysis of 28 food products (mostly CBD oil) in Germany containing hemp extract as an ingredient found that 10 products (36%) contained THC above the lowest level known to cause adverse effects (2.5 mg/day).(95)

CBD balances the immune system. That means it can calm an overactive immune system to support health by lowering the activity of immune cells known as T-cells.(8) CBD is also known to increase the number of natural killer (NK) cells.(8) These NK cells act like soldiers that go after and kill unwanted invaders in the body. Unlike most immune cells, NK cells have an interesting property: they can identify a stressed cell even if no antibodies to a particular virus is present. This leads to a faster immune response. Other immune cells aren't able to detect and destroy infected cells that don't have an antibody marker. This gives NK cells a definite advantage.

A large part of our immune system is located in our gut thanks to what's known as the gut-associated lymphoid tissues or GALT for short. Immune cells in GALT are able to recognize unwanted organisms, begin an immune response, and flag cells with markers known as antigens that help the immune system go after unhealthy cells. The gut microbiota, the microorganisms that reside in our intestines, interact with GALT to support a healthy immune system.

CBD can support a healthy inflammatory response and balance in the intestines.(96) The intestinal immune response then remains strong and supports the body's immune response as a whole.(96)

CBD can also maintain lung and respiratory health. It supports a healthy inflammatory response in the lungs of animals, maintains markers of lung health, while promoting healthy lung function.(97)

It's noteworthy that CBD use can also result in a calm mood and an increased ability to deal with occasional stress. Stress is known to wreak havoc on our immune systems.

Pharmaceuticals

Researchers have found some oral medications that may help in the treatment and potentially prevention of COVID-19. These include chloroquine and hydroxychloroquine.(98) Based upon in-vitro studies of the SARS coronavirus, nitazoxanide may also be an effective drug. (99) Protease inhibitors, particularly the combination of lopinavir and ritonavir, that have shown promise in other coronaviruses (SARS, MERS) are also showing potential to decrease disease severity and duration in COVID-19. (100)

Hydroxychloroquine, Chloroquine and COVID-19

Hydrochloroquine (HCQ) is an old malaria treatment approved by the FDA in 1955 and now also approved for treating lupus and rheumatoid arthritis. I took this medication while in medical school for malaria.

Chloroquine and HCQ have anti-viral activity against SARS-CoV-2 by preventing the virus attaching to host cells, theoretically making infected people less contagious, and it should reduce hospitalizations and deaths.

Bud was fortunate that his doctors started HCQ along with vitamin C during his hospitalization.

While we wait for placebo-controlled studies, this is a treatment that should be strongly considered. It may also be appropriate to start early when symptoms are mild, especially for our front-line health care workers and others in high-risk jobs where a lot of contact with infected people is likely.

Source: Cortegiani A, Ingoglia G, Ippolito M, et al. A systematic review on the efficacy and safety of chloroquine for the treatment of COVID-19. J Crit Care. 2020 Mar 10. pii: S0883-9441(20)30390-7. [Epub ahead of print.] doi: 10.1016/j.jcrc.2020.03.005

The information in this book is educational and Informational only: IT IS NOT MEDICAL ADVICE. It is not intended to diagnose or treat. No pharmaceutical or dietary supplement has been proven in long-term placebo-controlled studies to treat or prevent COVID-19.

STORIES

BUD

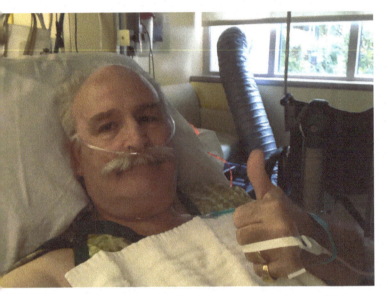

Bud on day 17 (March 29th) of hospitalization – thankfully avoided the ventilator and starting to recover.

My friend Bud is in his mid 60's, a jovial happy man who would give you the shirt of his back if you needed it.

By text message, he shared with me from his ICU hospital bed, his journey with COVID-19.

March 29, 2020: "Two weeks ago I was pretty sure I was a dead man at any moment. They wanted to put me on a life support ventilator. I fought it because most who go on the ventilator never live. They wanted to do it to prevent not having time to perform the insertion. I said no, if I'm conscious I have a chance to fight for my life. For the next several days they asked me if I was ready at least three or more times. I said no. With very little breath I fought. The prayers of so many and God will save me. I'm forever grateful. God bless."

Bud no doubt made the right choice, scary as it was. One study has shown that mechanical ventilation, and the increased pressures that are used are directly responsible for some of the lung damage.(101)

For Bud, this whole COVID-19 nightmare started a little over 2 weeks prior, when he got sick during the night of March 13 while on vacation to celebrate his 45th wedding anniversary at the Oregon coast in their 5th wheel trailer. By the next day (March 14) he had a full day of fever a 102.7. His wife, Gayle, called the hot line Sunday March 15 and was told since they were at the coast to stay put and call back in a few days if the fever persists.

Bud recalled: "I became too ill to hitch my 5th wheel to come home so we stayed put until Wednesday (March 18th) when I started to feel even worse. 'We need to go now' I told Gayle, so I struggled with my breathing and got us on the road. They [the clinic] wanted a conference call with us so I pulled over for about 20 minutes. Before we got back home, they called and said to come as fast as I could to Beaverton Clinic. I dropped the trailer at that point and Gayle drove me. They checked me over and sent me to the hospital by ambulance. The nurse looked at the report from the clinic in Beaverton. The oxygen level was 83% and was on the way down from there. God got us home from Astoria that day."

It was two days later, a week after Bud's symptoms started and two days after he was hospitalized, that I learned of his situation. This was the motivation to write this book.

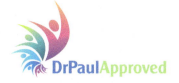

I reached out by text message in hopes that he was well enough to respond. He did! "I'm on oxygen. The fever is controlled by Advil. I have zero energy and a very dry cough. They started the malaria plan (chloroquine) for the next 5 days." As a physician, I'm aware that sometimes other doctors can allow a treatment that they consider experimental if it is thought it might have a chance of helping. I asked Bud to see if they would allow some vitamin C, melatonin and CBD on a compassionate use basis. In medicine we are moved by compassion so I hoped that might work.

On Monday, March 23 I sent him quick text: "You are in my prayers. How were the last 24 hours? Love Dr. Paul."

Bud responded: "A struggle for oxygen is a real issue. Fatigue. My ability to sleep is a challenge and on a liquid diet. I'm alive. Everyday has to be a gift from God. I'm worried about Gayle." That's Bud! On his potential last breath and worried about his dear wife Gayle.

I reassured Bud we would look after Gayle and indeed had taken her supplies as she herself was ill with more GI symptoms. I inquired how much oxygen he was needing. "It's not stable," he replied, "If I have coughing episodes my oxygen can go from 88/92 down to below 80. I'm on high flow humidified oxygen 30L & 70%."

That evening his doctor had started vitamin C, 1,000 mg twice a day!

A message from Bud's son posted to a group of friends was not to bother him as he needed rest. I waited for what I thought would be bad news. He had already signed a DNR (Do Not Resuscitate).

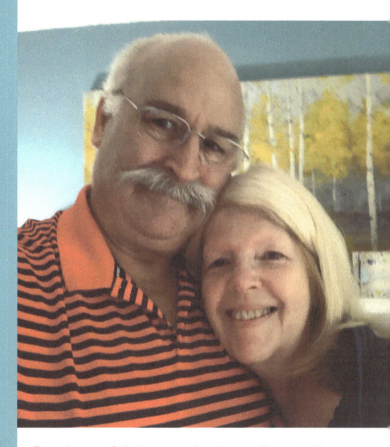

Imagine my delight to get the picture above with the message "God bless you my friend. I'm getting stronger daily. Thank God. I'm so blessed by God and awesome people in my life. Love you all."

On March 31, 2020, 18 days after his symptoms started, Bud was discharged to finish his recovery at home.

Not able to stand it any longer I reached out thinking that if he was starting to turn the corner at this point without being intubated that he actually had good chances of beating this thing.

Bud's first day home with his wife. He shared an image of his pulse ox at 97% on April 1, 2020.

NEW ORLEANS ER DOCTOR SHARES IT LIKE IT IS! CENSORED

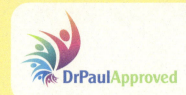

Anonymous - this has since been removed from Facebook

FOR MY MEDICAL PEOPLE, from a friend who worked in New Orleans: "I am an ER MD in New Orleans. Class of 98. Every one of my colleagues have now seen several hundred COVID-19 patients and this is what I think I know. Clinical course is predictable. 2-11 days after exposure (day 5 on average) flu-like symptoms start.

Common are fever, headache, dry cough, myalgias (back pain), nausea without vomiting, abdominal discomfort with some diarrhea, loss of smell, anorexia, fatigue.

Day 5 of symptoms- increased SOB, and bilateral viral pneumonia from direct viral damage to lung parenchyma.

Day 10- Cytokine storm leading to acute ARDS and multiorgan failure. You can literally watch it happen in a matter of hours. 81% mild symptoms, 14% severe symptoms requiring hospitalization, 5% critical. Patient presentation is varied. Patients are coming in hypoxic (even 75%) without dyspnea.

I have seen COVID-19 patients present with encephalopathy, renal failure from dehydration, DKA. I have seen bilateral interstitial pneumonia on the x-ray of the asymptomatic shoulder dislocation or on the CT's of the (respiratory) asymptomatic polytrauma patient. Essentially if they are in my ER, they have it.

Seen three positive flu swabs in 2 weeks and all three had COVID-19 as well. Somehow this ***** has told all other disease processes to get out of town.

China reported 15% cardiac involvement. I have seen 19 patients present with myocarditis, pericarditis, new onset CHF and new onset atrial fibrillation. I still order a troponin, but no cardiologist will treat no matter what the number in a suspected COVID-19 patient.

Even our non COVID-19 STEMIs [ST-Elevation Myocardial Infarction, a very serious type of heart attack] at all of our facilities are getting TPA [Tissue plasminogen activator] in the ED [Emergency Department] and rescue PCI at 60 minutes only if TPA fails.

Diagnostic CXR- bilateral interstitial pneumonia (anecdotally starts most often in the RLL [right lower lobe] so bilateral on [chest x-ray] CXR is not required). The hypoxia does not correlate with the CXR findings. Their lungs do not sound bad.

Keep your stethoscope in your pocket and evaluate with your eyes and pulse ox.

Labs - WBC low, Lymphocytes low, platelets lower than their normal, Procalcitonin normal in 95% CRP and Ferritin elevated most often. CPK, D-Dimer, LDH, Alk Phos/AST/ALT commonly elevated. Notice D-Dimer -I would be very careful about CT PE these patients for their hypoxia. The patients receiving IV contrast are going into renal failure and on the vent sooner.

Basically, if you have bilateral pneumonia with normal to low WBC, lymphopenia, normal procalcitonin, elevated CRP and ferritin - you have COVID-19 and do not need a nasal swab to tell you that. A ratio of absolute neutrophil count to absolute lymphocyte count greater than 3.5 may be the highest predictor of poor outcome.

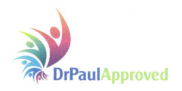

The UK is automatically intubating these patients for expected outcomes regardless of their clinical presentation. An elevated Interleukin-6 (IL6) is an indicator of their cytokine storm. If this is elevated watch these patients closely with both eyes. Other factors that appear to be predictive of poor outcomes are thrombocytopenia and LFTs 5x upper limit of normal.

Disposition: I had never discharged multifocal pneumonia before. Now I personally do it 12-15 times a shift. 2 weeks ago, we were admitting anyone who needed supplemental oxygen. Now we are discharging with oxygen if the patient is comfortable and oxygenating above 92% on nasal cannula.

We have contracted with a company that sends a paramedic to their home twice daily to check on them and record a pulse ox. We know many of these patients will bounce back but if it saves a bed for a day, we have accomplished something.

Obviously, we are fearful some won't make it back.

We are a small community hospital. Our 22 bed ICU and now a 4 bed Endoscopy suite are all COVID-19. All of these patients are intubated except one. 75% of our floor beds have been cohorted into COVID-19 wards and are full.

We are averaging 4 rescue intubations a day on the floor. We now have 9 vented patients in our ER transferred down from the floor after intubation.

Luckily, we are part of a larger hospital group. Our main teaching hospital repurposed space to open 50 new COVID-19 ICU beds this past Sunday so these numbers are with significant decompression.

Today those 50 beds are full.

They are opening 30 more by Friday. But even with the "lockdown", our AI models are expecting a 200-400% increase in COVID-19 patients by 4/4/2020.

Treatment Supportive

Worldwide, 86% of COVID19 patients that go on a vent die. Seattle reporting 70%. Our hospital has had 5 deaths and one patient who was extubated. Extubation happens on day 10 per the Chinese and day 11 per Seattle.

Plaquenil which has weak ACE2 blockade doesn't appear to be a savior of any kind in our patient population. Theoretically, it may have some prophylactic properties but so far it is difficult to see the benefit to our hospitalized patients, but we are using it and the studies will tell. With Plaquenil's potential QT prolongation and liver toxic effects (both particularly problematic in COVID-19 patients).

I am no longer selectively prescribing this medication as I stated on a previous post. We are also using Azithromycin but are intermittently running out of IV.

Do not give these patient's standard sepsis fluid resuscitation. Be very judicious with the fluids as it hastens their respiratory decompensation.

The information in this book is educational and Informational only: IT IS NOT MEDICAL ADVICE. It is not intended to diagnose or treat. No pharmaceutical or dietary supplement has been proven in long-term placebo-controlled studies to treat or prevent COVID-19.

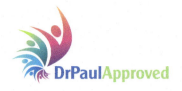

Outside the DKA and renal failure dehydration, leave them dry. Proning vented patients significantly helps oxygenation. Even self proning the ones on nasal cannula helps.

Vent settings - Usual ARDS stuff, low volume, permissive hypercapnia, etc. Except for Peep of 5 will not do. Start at 14 and you may go up to 25 if needed. Do not use Bipap- it does not work well and is a significant exposure risk with high levels of aerosolized virus to you and your staff. Even after a cough or sneeze this virus can aerosolized up to 3 hours. The same goes for nebulizer treatments. Use MDI. You can give 8-10 puffs at one time of an albuterol MDI. Use only if wheezing which isn't often with COVID-19. If you have to give a nebulizer must be in a negative pressure room; and if you can, instruct the patient on how to start it after you leave the room.

Do not use steroids, it makes this worse. Push out to your urgent cares to stop their usual practice of steroid shots for their URI/bronchitis.

We are currently out of Versed, Fentanyl, and intermittently Propofol. Get the dosing of Precedex and Nimbex back in your heads.

One of my colleagues who is a 31 yo old female who graduated residency last May with no health problems and normal BMI is out with the symptoms and an SaO2 of 92%. She will be the first of many.

I PPE best I have. I do wear a MaxAir PAPR the entire shift. I do not take it off to eat or drink during the shift. I undress in the garage and go straight to the shower. My wife and kids fled to her parents outside Hattiesburg. The stress and exposure at work coupled with the isolation at home is trying. But everyone is going through something right now. Everyone is scared; patients and employees. But we are the leaders of that emergency room. Be nice to your nurses and staff. Show by example how to tackle this crisis head on.

Good luck to us all."

IMPORTANT LESSONS From our anonymous ER Doctor.

1. Symptoms start 2-11 days after exposure (day 5 on average)
2. Flu like symptoms then fever, headache, dry cough, myalgias (back pain), nausea without vomiting, abdominal discomfort with some diarrhea, loss of smell, anorexia, fatigue.
3. Day 5 of symptoms - increased SOB (shortness of breath),
4. Pneumonia from direct viral damage to lung parenchyma.
5. Day 10 - cytokine storm leading to acute ARDS and multiorgan failure
6. You can have low oxygen without obvious pneumonia on exam or x-ray
7. Can have oxygen as low as 75% without major symptoms
8. WBC low, lymphocytes low, platelets low
9. Oxygen at home a reasonable approach unless you absolutely need intubation
10. 70% - 86% of the intubated die (I haven't checked all sources on this statistic). If true, Bud was wise to battle on without intubation, which was offered to him at least 3 times.
11. Being dehydrated (within reason) is a good thing (your lungs don't fill up with fluid)
12. Avoid steroids.
13. Those working with COVID-19 patients: keep your whole body protection on the entire shift, taking it on and off to eat likely increases risk. Maybe work a bit dehydrated so you don't have to use the bathroom, eat and drink when you get home!

SUMMARY – PUTTING THINGS IN PERSPECTIVE

THOUGHTS

Many doctors and healthcare workers are literally dying themselves, making heroic sacrifices trying to apply a broken model of health care to the COVID-19 pandemic. They simply don't know what they don't know and are doing the best they can with what they know. Of course, you want to be on the ventilator if you would die without it! Yes, we need modern medicine.

I am very impressed with their bravery and self-sacrifice. Everyone who knowingly cares for anyone infected with COVID-19 coronavirus does so at some risk. We have physicians coming out of retirement to help, knowing they are at the highest risk due to their age.

That said, I'm heartbroken that so few understand that the solution for most is as simple as taking massive doses of vitamin C. Most physicians stand by and watch their patients die rather than use ascorbic acid (vitamin C). Intravenous vitamin C, when available, should be used for those who are sickest. The rest of us can use oral vitamin C. As we get sicker (if we do) we start ramping up the dose to bowel tolerance (causes severe diarrhea at high doses). I'm learning that the sicker you are the more vitamin C you can tolerate. If I were struggling with a COVID-19 infection, I would ramp my dose up to as much as 100,000 mg of oral vitamin C a day, dividing it into doses as frequent as every 10 - 15 minutes if it was tolerated and I was heading toward a ventilator. I suspect 1,000 mg several times a day is enough to keep you from getting sick.

Now to put this COVID-19 coronavirus infection in perspective. Each year most of us get a common cold or "flu." Coronaviruses have been one of the more than 100 viruses that can cause the common cold or flu like symptoms. Each year up until 2020, for decades now, our CDC officials have lumped all respiratory infections and deaths into one category and attribute them to the "flu." If we dumb it down to "the flu is killing all these people," when it actually is over 100 viruses and numerous bacterial infections or a combination of these along with the patient's underlying health conditions, we can create a mind set in the population that says, "I need to get a flu shot!" But realize this – the flu shot covers just 3 - 4 strains of influenza and does nothing against the hundreds of other agents that may be causing your "flu." When they do roll out a coronavirus vaccine, it will have had no long-term safety studies and will be a huge experiment with possible disastrous long-term consequences.

We are always reminded of the flu pandemic of 1918. In that one flu season about 20 million died worldwide. What we forget is that this pandemic occurred during and after World War I, which had raged from 1914-1918, killing about 10 million soldiers. Was it a lack of vaccines that caused those 20 million to die of the flu? Or was it that years of massive stress and malnutrition had so weakened our immune systems that we were particularly vulnerable?

The information in this book is educational and Informational only: IT IS NOT MEDICAL ADVICE. It is not intended to diagnose or treat. No pharmaceutical or dietary supplement has been proven in long-term placebo-controlled studies to treat or prevent COVID-19.

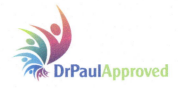

The modern set-up for a pandemic is exactly what we have today. Our population is generally more stressed than at any time in the past. Stress as seemingly insignificant as the excessive amount of time spent on that little handheld computer we call a phone, social media and 24/7 bad news are compounded by war for many parts of the world, horrible nutrition in the form of sugar and packaged foods that do nothing to boost the immune system or provide nutrients required for health in our bodies. Our gut immunity has been destroyed by the herbicide glyphosate. And the 5-G being rolled out across the world is suspected of harming our immune system.(102) Our world is basically primed for such an epidemic.

What we need to survive this and the future novel viral infections that will certainly come along, is not a vaccine, but healthy immune systems, healthy habits, real immune-boosting nutritious food. Given the impossibility of those strategies for so many people, we need appropriate supplementation of key immune-boosting nutrients. Perhaps above all else, we need a mindset that is fitness and wellness focused, with special attention to reducing stress.

Since we now have the technology to identify actual viral protein sequences, we are able to identify the mutations in the strains that circulate each year. Earlier in this book I showed you the similarity of the various coronaviruses, and it is interesting to look at the mutations over the decades for the flu virus. From the 1918 Spanish flu that killed so many back then all the way to 2008 you can see the relationships year to year. Something unexplainable seems to have happened in 2009. That strain, shown below in the bottom right of the diagram, is most like the 1918 Spanish flu virus on the bottom left. How does a virus jump backwards, erasing decades of mutations, to resemble what it was like almost 100 years earlier?

The diagram below shows the relationship of flu viruses through the past century.

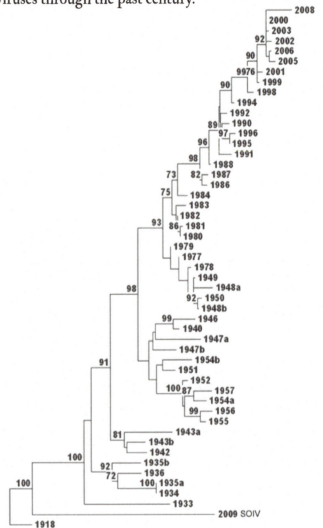

"Phylogenetic analysis of the HA1 of H1N1 influenza viruses. Phylogenetic tree constructed using the neighbor-joining method and bootstrap analysis (n = 500) to determine the best-fitting tree for the HA1 region of the HA gene. Selected, relevant strains of the H1N1 subtype are listed by year of isolation. Small case "a" and "b" designate when two distinct strains co-circulated in the same year. Bootstrap values ≥ 70% are shown at branchpoints."

Source: https://bmcinfectdis.biomedcentral.com/articles/10.1186/1471-2334-10-5#Fig2

Whether this happened by accident or was an intentional release for some malicious reason, we will never know. What does seem certain, given the novel (new) COVID-19 infection, and this example of the Spanish Flu mysteriously returning in 2009 is that we will likely see more such events.

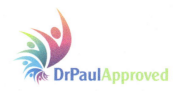

HOW DO WE DEFEND OURSELVES

I'd propose that it is past time that we take our personal care and support of your own immune system seriously. You will either have a robust immune system that you can boost with tools like those I'm mentioning in this book, or you will look to outside forces to come to your rescue with drugs and vaccines.

I was finishing high school and starting college in the mid 1970s when the Swine Flu outbreak occurred. I wasn't vaccinated, nor was I aware there was a vaccine being pushed for it at that time. I'm grateful I wasn't vaccinated as it turned out to be a huge mistake. FDA documents stated the flu shot could result in "some minor side effects -tenderness in the arm, low fever, tiredness" and that these effects "will occur in less than 4% of (vaccinated) adults. Serious reactions from flu vaccines are very rare."

Serious side effects of Swine Flu vaccine forced the federal immunization program to a halt. So much for safety claims. When asked the question, "what can be done to prevent an epidemic?", the answer you will undoubtedly hear is that "the only preventive action we can take is to develop a vaccine to immunize the public against the virus. This will prevent the virus from spreading."

The immunization program for Swine Flu was abruptly halted and yet there was still no epidemic. If vaccination was the only defense, tens of millions of Americans should have died! That of course did not happen.

From the diagram above you can see there was another interesting gap in the strains since the 1918 Spanish Flu, with yearly mutations until the 1950s then a jump of almost 30 years.

We had Zika, then Ebola, and there will be many more. During an infection crisis, quarantine can be a vital tool to preventing the spread of most infectious diseases. It is interesting to note that herd immunity, what some call community immunity, is strongest when the population develops natural immunity, which is exactly what has happened since the beginning of time. We likely will have massive herd immunity from the COVID-19 infections as they appear to be reaching a large percentage of the population. While I'm not a public health official, and I certainly am not advocating for this because we just don't have enough information yet, I suspect our best approach going forward will be to allow the young and healthy to get the COVID-19 infections, and support them with the key immune-boosting nutrients. They will then provide the community immunity to protect the elderly and more vulnerable among us. If a relatively safe and effective vaccine can be developed, then it should be given to the elderly and high-risk individuals while we continue to let the natural immunity expand among the young and the healthy.

Don't fall for the trap where your fear that COVID-19 will kill you leads you to accept a dangerous vaccine, thinking it is the only thing that will save you. Neither are true. COVID-19 won't kill you (we will lose some of the most vulnerable and that is very sad) and the vaccine likely won't save you.

The information in this book is educational and Informational only: IT IS NOT MEDICAL ADVICE. It is not intended to diagnose or treat. No pharmaceutical or dietary supplement has been proven in long-term placebo-controlled studies to treat or prevent COVID-19.

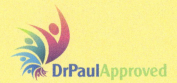

Our long history with vaccine efforts would suggest that natural immunity for these types of viral infections is the way to go. The truth of the matter, when it comes to vaccines, is that there is a balance of risk and benefit. When the data is robust as to the risks and benefits, which it rarely is, then the decisions would be easy. Sadly, due to the lack of real placebo-controlled studies that are long term (years), we are always left having to guess which is better or worse, natural risks or the vaccine risks? Natural immunity or vaccine-induced immunity and vaccine side effects?

The heroes of the COVID-19 2020 pandemic will be those who put themselves in danger, developed natural immunity that will likely be lasting, and thus offer a shield of protection for the rest of us.

Let us make sure we are testing for immunity before giving anyone a vaccine, as we don't want to inadvertently destroy those who are actually offering us the best protection against COVID-19 next season and going forward.

Let us honor informed consent that gives every human the right to bodily integrity. We should insist on the precautionary principle that would have us need to prove long-term safety before offering a potentially dangerous vaccine to an unsuspecting public who are undoubtedly now going to have PTSD at just the word "coronavirus" or "COVID."

Remember, we have handled past coronaviruses just fine and we will conquer this one too!

It is a healthy body, healthy mind, healthy spirit and most importantly a healthy immune system that will protect us going forward.

It is now time for a paradigm shift.

It is time to get back to the basics of eating organic (if possible) fruits and vegetables, avoiding immune-destroying sugar and processed foods, significantly reducing stress, exercising, getting our sleep, and reaching out to help our fellow humans, living in a loving and nurturing community. We were never intended for isolation.

If you have suffered the loss of a loved one, you are most certainly grieving. Embrace the grief, get help and allow yourself to work through it.

I suspect most of us are also experiencing what has been called anticipatory grief. In a very real way, everything is changing and fast! We wonder if the life we had become used to will ever return back to "normal."

Anticipatory grief is that feeling we get about what the future holds when we're uncertain. While it usually centers on death, we feel it when a loved one gets a dire diagnosis, but also when we are simply anticipating a storm coming. There's the sense that something bad is out there. With the coronavirus it is confusing, since we can't see it. Our sense of safety is shattered.

To combat this anticipatory grief and find balance, focus your thoughts on those you love and on positive things in your life and make a daily habit of writing down and expressing gratitude. Call or communicate positively with your friends, family and loved ones. If you find yourself future-tripping in fear, come back to the present. Let go of what you cannot control.

The Serenity Prayer

God, grant me the serenity,
To accept the things I cannot change,
To change the things I can
And the wisdom to know the difference"

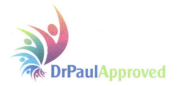

THE RUSH FOR A VACCINE

By the time the COVID-19 pandemic of 2020 is a year behind us it is likely that this virus will have been the deadliest worldwide infection in the past century. Historians will compare it to smallpox, the Spanish Flu, and the great plagues, but there has certainly been nothing like it for those of us living today. Our modern connected world, where so many can jump on an airplane and travel anywhere, has enabled COVID-19 to spread around the entire globe. Our ability to communicate and see in real time what is going on around the globe makes this pandemic unique also.

They say ignorance is bliss. Our innocence has been shattered. In times like these, we look for a savior. In times like these, there is not only great opportunity, but great danger.

What risks would you be willing to take in hopes that there is a cure or a way to prevent future infection with COVID-19?

You can already hear the messaging about vaccines. They are coming to save the world. Just hang on a little longer.

I'm not saying vaccines are good or bad. Vaccines can most certainly boost the immunity against a given pathogen. Since I was in medical school in the early 1980s when AIDS was beginning, they have been working on an AIDS vaccine – without success. I suspect, however, that this time will be different. This time, if our scientists have it right as to the exact cause of COVID-19 being the SARS-CoV-2, then they are targeting a specific pathogen, and chances of getting a vaccine that will boost immunity against SARS-CoV-2 are good. What is unknown and cannot be known is at what cost? How much collateral damage will the vaccines cause. Usually vaccines harm your immune system by creating autoimmune problems and sometimes the vaccines create a situation where you are less able to fight the new strains that inevitably appear in subsequent years.

Natural immunity is always better. Dr James Crowe at Vanderbilt University reported live with Dana Perino April 2 2020 that patients who had COVID-19 and recovered have a very robust immune response and that a couple months out, they are harvesting these antibodies and creating more that can be used to treat active COVID-19 infections.

A robust immune response that lasts!

That is what you get with natural infection. These patients being treated with antibodies, while good at the time, will not have lasting protection. Those vaccinated with the coming experimental vaccines will be just that – a grand experiment – with each coming season of COVID-19 and the mutant viruses that come from it representing potential disaster.

The information in this book is educational and Informational only: IT IS NOT MEDICAL ADVICE. It is not intended to diagnose or treat. No pharmaceutical or dietary supplement has been proven in long-term placebo-controlled studies to treat or prevent COVID-19.

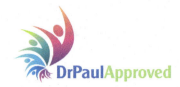

HERD IMMUNITY

Herd immunity, sometimes called community immunity, is the concept that the herd (our population) will be protected from a disease when a large enough percentage of the population has had the disease and is immune.

The term herd immunity originated from the natural childhood diseases where every few years enough children were born who had not had measles or chickenpox that the illness could take hold in the population. There would be months or a year of infections and the herd (population) would once again be protected.

For diseases for which we have a vaccine, it has been used to say that when a high enough percentage of the population has been vaccinated against a given disease, that the population is protected from outbreaks. For measles, it is claimed that 95% of the population needs to be vaccinated. The reality is that many adults under the age of 64 (born after 1957) no longer have measles protection, so that the actual rate of protection in the population is likely more like 60% - 70% and yet we still have had no real issue with measles the past decade in the USA. Those of us born before 1957 are still immune to measles because natural infection is known to give lifelong protection.

My vote is always for natural immune protection if possible. The Holy Grail for pharma is the opposite – create a vaccine that everyone wants and then get it mandated, and without liability if anything goes wrong. The feeding frenzy is on!

Those my age and older (I'm in my 60s) remember getting all the childhood diseases and even intentionally exposing ourselves, to get the immunity.

A kind of natural immunization if you will. This worked well for almost all diseases. A nice aspect of this natural immunity, acquired through natural infection, was that the children, who rarely died and for whom the illnesses tended to be mild or at least more tolerable, would boost the immunity of the older children and adults who already had antibodies. Natural infection acted like a vaccine booster.

For those diseases that now have vaccines, we have discovered new challenges. Vaccine-induced immunity is not as robust and typically wanes over time. Most organisms when exposed to the vaccine will over time naturally select changes that enable them to bypass the vaccine. These mutant strains become the predominant ones since the vaccine shuts off the viability of the strain for which there is a vaccine.

KEYS TO A SAFE VACCINE

1. It is specific against just the organism to avoid molecular mimicry that triggers an autoimmune response where your immune system attacks you.
2. It does not contain toxic ingredients that themselves trigger health problems.
3. It is safety tested with a saline placebo arm to the trials.
4. Safety testing includes long-term (years) of follow-up looking at all health outcomes.

There are no vaccines that meet the simple standards of safety in the box above, since most do not use saline as the placebo or don't have a placebo arm at all. None of the safety trials are long term and they don't look at all health outcomes. The current, first vaccine trial in humans against SARS-CoV-2, does not have a placebo arm to it. Why? It would be so easy to have an equal number of people receive a saline injection!

The information in this book is educational and Informational only: IT IS NOT MEDICAL ADVICE. It is not intended to diagnose or treat. No pharmaceutical or dietary supplement has been proven in long-term placebo-controlled studies to treat or prevent COVID-19.

Let me answer my own question. If 5 of the 45 extremely healthy individuals (we always exclude anyone with any underlying health issues when selecting people to run vaccine experiments on) die over the next 5 years after getting the new COVID vaccine, and another 10 go on to develop debilitating autoimmune issues, it can be claimed that this was to be expected. So there were no unexpected side effects. That would be a 10% death rate in young healthy subjects and a 20% chronic disease rate. If we had a saline placebo group who had no deaths and 1 person went on to develop autoimmune issues we could then see that the vaccine in this trial would be more dangerous than a COVID-19 infection.

Given that example, putting high-risk individuals in quarantine and intentionally getting all the young and healthy people exposed to develop natural immunity would in fact result in better herd immunity. Natural infection would actually be the best solution – not a vaccine.

DO WE HAVE ANY RECENT EXAMPLES OF FAST-TRACKING VACCINE DEVELOPEMNT?

The vaccine rushed to market for H1N1 went on to increase miscarriages in pregnant women in the USA(103) and provoked a massive spike in narcolepsy. (104)(105)(106)(107)(108) In Australia one in every 110 vaccinated children had a febrile seizure.(109) The challenge in most vaccine studies is that the side effect data is hidden from view and companies profiting from these vaccines have no incentive to share bad outcomes.

With massive profits to be made, biotech companies are racing for the jackpot. There are at least 35 COVID-19 vaccines in the pipeline.(110)

The PREP Act (Public Readiness and Emergency Preparedness Act) protects manufacturers from all liability for vaccines for COVID-19 as this has been declared a public health emergency.(111) This basically is a blank check to Big Pharma and biotech companies.

PATHOGENIC PRIMING - Warning to those making vaccines for COVID-19

New study results point to the very high likelihood that vaccination against SARS-CoV-2 would lead to autoimmunity against specific tissues. The tissues match those we see issues with in COVID-19 - but also point to a large number and % of potentially targeted human immune system proteins.

Perhaps we should be thinking about COVID-19 disease caused by the SARS-CoV-2 virus, as an autoimmune disorder. This should guide our treatment approaches and should absolutely require animal safety studies and long term follow-up for any vaccine being considered. Author J Lyons-Weiler concludes, "

SARS-CoV-2 has some unexplained pathogenic features that might be related to the table of putative pathogenic priming peptides. Exposure to these specific peptides - via either infection or vaccination - might prime patients for increased risk of enhanced pathogenicity during future exposure due either to future pandemic or outbreaks or via universal vaccination programs. While the mechanisms [of] pathogenesis of COVID-19 are still poorly understood, the morbidity and mortality of SARS has been extensively studied. Thus, the involvement of pathogenic priming in re-infection by COVID-19 is a theoretical possibility; of course no vaccine against SARS-CoV-2 has yet been tested in animals and therefore we do not yet know if pathogenic priming is in fact expected. Such studies should be undertaken before use of any vaccine against SARS-CoV-2 is used in humans."

The article also points to specific epitopes that should be excluded from any SARS-CoV-2/COVID-19 vaccine to avoid induction of autoimmunity. Such a step might reduce the risk of disease enhancement via pathogenic priming.

J. Lyons-Weiler, Pathogenic Priming Likely Contributes to Serious and Critical Illness and Mortality in COVID-19 via Autoimmunity, Journal of Translational Autoimmunity, https://doi.org/10.1016/j.jtauto.2020.100051.

CONFLICTS OF INTEREST

The FDA receives 45% of its annual budget from industry.(112) The World Health Organization (WHO) gets half its budget from private sources, Pharma and its allied foundations.(113) CDC is a vaccine company that owns 56 vaccine patents,(114) and buys and distributes $4.6 billion in vaccines annually through the Vaccines for Children program which represents over 40% of its total budget.(115)

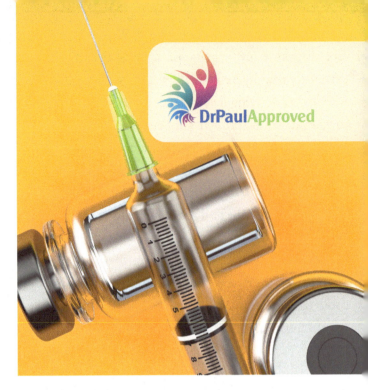

WOULD I RECOMMEND A VACCINE FOR COVID-19?

Sure, if it is properly designed and long-term safety-tested and data suggests it will be highly effective, AND if there is a need. Those already immune from natural infection should NOT be vaccinated!

The challenge I see will be the lack of proper clinical trials. The vaccine industry already has a track record of not doing proper studies that would show side effects. Think about it. Are you going to invest millions and reduce the chances your product will be acceptable by doing properly designed studies that show problems with your product? Of course not.

For those who are longing for a Pharma savior, there will be plenty lining up for your money and adoration.

For those inclined to wait and get more data, there will be enormous pressure on you to roll up your sleeve or else! I worry that our post 2020 COVID-19 world will look very different.

Travel to many or most countries will likely require either proof of immunity or proof of vaccination. If we get the testing for the antibodies (IgM for current or recent infection and IgG for evidence of immunity) we will know if we are at risk or not. During the next round, wouldn't it be nice to know that the health care professionals working on you and the workers in homes for the elderly are immune and thus cannot give you the virus?

We clearly need more data.

Some good news: recent research submitted for publication ("Reinfection could not occur in SARS-CoV-2 infected rhesus macaques") showed that these monkeys, once infected, developed lasting immunity and when challenged with the same SARS-CoV-2 virus did not develop COVID-19 infections.(116) This would bode well for the idea of testing everyone for evidence of antibodies against this virus and if we have them we are likely immune and certainly would not need or want a vaccine.

IS IT TIME FOR A PARADIGM SHIFT?

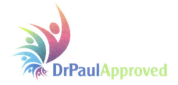

We live in a time where chronic diseases are killing most of us, not infections. In our battle to fight infections, we have created so much collateral damage that developmental delays in children, chronic diseases, allergies, asthma, eczema and autoimmune conditions now affect most of us. Do you remember a time when no one you knew had any health issues? I do.

Pasteur, the father of the germ theory, proposed that "germs are bad" and they are the cause of disease and ill health. And that the solution to both treating and preventing illness was to kill them. Basically that germs (virus, bacteria, etc.) cause illness which is the foundation of Western Medicine, which led to over use of vaccinations, antibiotics and other antimicrobials. In the process we have altered the biome (the balance of the healthy organisms in and on our bodies).

Pasteur's bitter rival, Bechamp, advocated not the killing of germs but rather the cultivation of health through diet, hygiene and healthy lifestyle practices like getting enough fresh air and exercise. The idea being that a strong immune system and good tissue quality (or "terrain" as Bechamp called it), prevented germs from causing harm. We now know that our microbiome and biome are exactly what we need to be healthy, to have a robust immune system. Only when a person's health starts to decline (due to personal neglect and poor lifestyle choices) do they become victim to infections.

Pasteur – the father of the germ theory – last words were: "Le microbe n'est rien, le terrain est tout."

(The microbe is nothing, the terrain is everything) By the end of his life he knew he had been wrong. It is high time we figure that out ourselves!

It is indeed time for a paradigm shift. Health and wellness will not come from a needle injected concoction, nor from a pharmaceutical drug. Health will return when we nurture our wonderful immune systems, give our bodies the healing, life-giving nutrients they need and guard against the stresses that break down our immune system.

FINAL THOUGHTS

Remember that once this storm is over, we will have a hard time remembering how we made it through, but make it through we shall. We may not even be sure the storm is over but one thing we can count on with certainty is that we won't be the same person we were going into this as when we come out on the other side.

My wish for you is that we all come out with greater compassion, more grateful for all that we do have, and acting more forgiving and loving with one another.

"Do not be daunted by the enormity of the world's grief. Do justly, now. Love mercy, now. Walk humbly, now. You are not obligated to complete the work, but neither are you free to abandon it." The Talmud

May we all approach each other and our world with kindness, love and humility.

There is a very high probability that the media has way overblown this. That is what the media loves to do!

This is a new virus. Being new it will infect some percentage of the population. What is that percentage? When we test a large segment of a population that data can direct us. OHSU (Oregon Health Sciences University) is the largest employer in Portland, Oregon. This is where most of the region's sickest patients end up. There are over 17,000 employees who treated over 300,000 patients last year. While most hospitals have kept their COVID-19 data a secret, OHSU is publicizing all of their COVID-19 data for all to see.(117) So how many at OHSU are hospitalized for COVID-19? As I write this on April 4th....SIX!

My good friend who works at the other major trauma center in Portland (Legacy Emanuel) reported to me that the hospital is a ghost town. There is almost nothing going on. The third largest hospital in Portland, where I go to see babies - empty! Almost no one is walking the halls. The tents outside the ER are empty. I don't see people lined up to be checked.

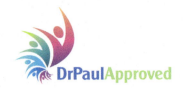

OHSU COVID-19 (Saturday, April 4)

39 COVID-19 cases to date:

20 inpatient/ED, 19 outpatient

33 tested positive at OHSU,

6 tested elsewhere and transferred to OHSU

Of 20 inpatient/ED patients: 12 discharged, 2 deceased, 6 remain in hospital

Oregon Health & Science University employees tested for COVID-19 to date: 1,253.

- 20 tested positive,
- 1,172 tested negative,
- 61 tests are pending.

Of all the employees tested only 20/1,253 were positive. That is 1.6% or 1 out of every 62 employees who have tested positive. Are Oregonians less vulnerable or is this the real picture when you actually do the testing! I'm guessing this is the real picture.

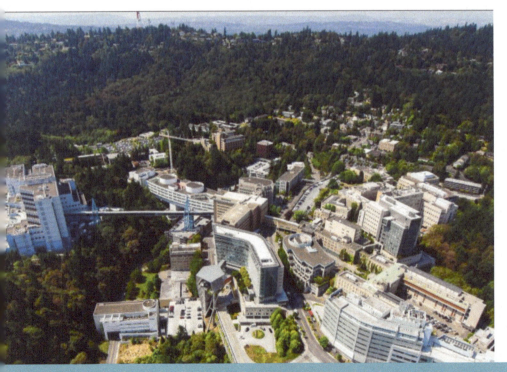

The information in this book is educational and Informational only: IT IS NOT MEDICAL ADVICE. It is not intended to diagnose or treat. No pharmaceutical or dietary supplement has been proven in long-term placebo-controlled studies to treat or prevent COVID-19.

For all of Oregon, looking at the graphic below, we can see that we seemed to have passed the peak already.

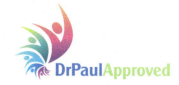

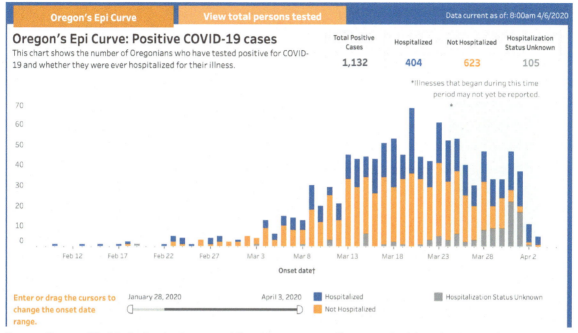

Source: Oregon Health Authority. https://public.tableau.com/profile/oregon.health.authority.covid.19#!/vizhome/OregonHealthAuthorityCOVID-19DataDashboard/COVID-19EPIConfirmed?:display_count=y&:toolbar=n&:origin=viz_share_link&:showShareOptions=false

Oregon's governor Kate Brown gave the shelter in place order on March 23. With the average incubation for COVID-19 being 5 days, we can see that the decline in cases had already largely played out before this order was given. By the time you read this, it may well be time for most of us to get back to work.

A good way to see if the country is actually coming out of this as predicted is to compare the death numbers being reported to the predictions. Here is a graph of predictions:

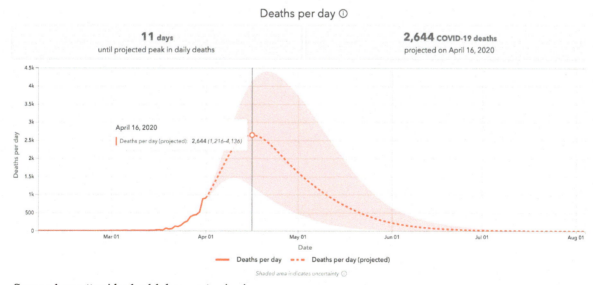

Source: https://covid19.healthdata.org/projections

The information in this book is educational and Informational only: IT IS NOT MEDICAL ADVICE. It is not intended to diagnose or treat. No pharmaceutical or dietary supplement has been proven in long-term placebo-controlled studies to treat or prevent COVID-19.

We will need the data like that which OHSU provided, on the rates of infection in the whole population, and better yet, the percentage of the population that developed immunity. The tests for COVID-19 only detect those infected at the time. What should inform our decisions going forward is what percentage of us are already immune. What if 80% of us were infected but had such minor infections that we never considered it could be COVID-19? What if most of us are already immune? What if this is a virus that can only take hold in those who are immunocompromised to begin with, those who have had previous flu shots, those exposed to the most glyphosate? We need to figure out the real risk factors so we can address them. Those same risk factors will undoubtedly come to play in the near future, but just with a different virus.

An important factor few are discussing is the push to identify this virus in all who die in hospitals. If you die of underlying conditions but happen to test positive for this coronavirus your death is being attributed to the virus. What about all the other viruses that are in your body at the time of death? We don't test for those! The presence of a virus at the time of death does not mean it was the cause of death. In my state of Oregon, where I now get the daily reports on each death, all 14 deaths (Oregon's 30th to 44th deaths) reported this past week had underlying health conditions. When we compare total deaths for the country and compare them to past years and past flu seasons, we will get a much better picture. If there is no substantial change in total deaths, it is likely that what has occurred is diagnostic substitution. We have merely changed the cause of death on the death certificate from complications of heart disease, diabetes or immunocompromised conditions to COVID-19.

I'd propose that you insist on knowing this information before agreeing to an experimental vaccine that has no long-term safety testing. At the very least you should insist on placebo controlled data that goes through the next season. Who will fare best in the winter flu season of 2020-2021? Those who developed natural immunity or those taking the experimental vaccines and the flu shots that have been shown to increase your risk of COVID-19?(118)

To Your Health. Blessings,
Dr. Paul

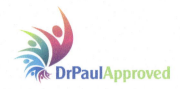

PLEASE HELP ME SAVE LIVES BY REVIEWING THIS BOOK

I wrote this book to save the lives of as many people as possible. You can help me in this quest by writing an honest review of the book on your favorite retailer's website. This will help other readers find it and obtain the knowledge they need to stay healthy.

With heartfelt thanks, Dr. Paul.

Guidelines for ER and Critical Care Doctors

Paul Marik, M.D. has compiled an **EVMS CRITICAL CARE COVID-19 MANAGEMENT PROTOCOL**. He is asking this to be distributed widely. It is brilliant and very important guidance for physicians caring for the sickest COVID Patients. Find it at evms.edu/covidcare.

DISCLAIMER

No statements in this book have been evaluated by the Food and Drug Administration. Nothing written, and no information within this book nor products mentioned are intended to diagnose, treat, cure or prevent any disease. This book is purely informational and educational. Anything you might learn should be reviewed by your personal physician.

The information in this book is educational and Informational only: IT IS NOT MEDICAL ADVICE. It is not intended to diagnose or treat. No pharmaceutical or dietary supplement has been proven in long-term placebo-controlled studies to treat or prevent COVID-19.

ABOUT THE AUTHOR
PAUL THOMAS, MD, ABAM, FAAP

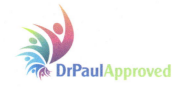

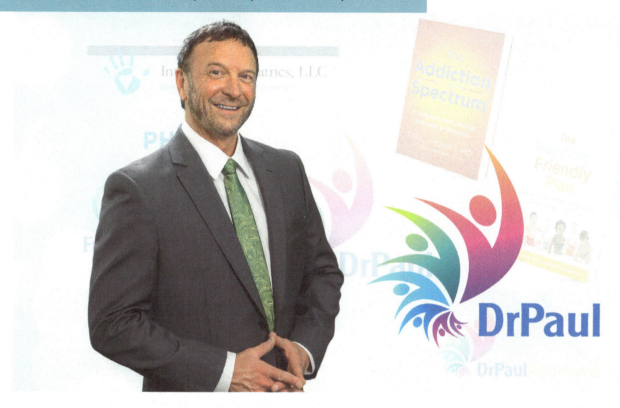

"The time has come to take our health and that of our children into our own hands." –
Dr. Paul Thomas

"Gone are the days when you could blindly follow your doctor's recommendations or count on your health plan or some government agency to put your best interests first. We owe it to ourselves and our children to remain constantly educated and informed so that we can make the best health decisions for ourselves and our families." –
Dr. Paul Thomas

Dr. Paul Thomas (affectionately known as "Dr. Paul") received his MD from Dartmouth Medical School in 1985. Dr. Paul is board-certified in Pediatrics and Addiction Medicine.

He has taught residents and medical students since 1988 and opened his own practice, Integrative Pediatrics, in 2008 where he currently serves over 15,000 patients in the Portland, Oregon area. Dr. Paul opened Fair Start, his medical detox clinic, in 2009, where he has helped over 1,000 patients wean off a wide range of opiates. He is the author of The Vaccine-Friendly Plan, published in 2016 by Ballantine Books. He is also author of The Addiction Spectrum – A Compassionate, Holistic Approach to Recovery, published by Harper One in 2018. In addition, he was host of The Addiction Summit, www.theaddictionsummit.com

Dr. Paul has over 1 million subscribers on his YouTube channel: https://www.youtube.com/user/paulthomasmd

Dr. Paul invites you to sign up for newsletters about keeping you and your family healthy, get important links and stay connected at:

www.DrPaulApproved.com

REFERENCES

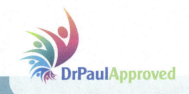

1. Wölfel R, Corman VM, Guggemos W, et al. Virological assessment of hospitalized cases of coronavirus disease 2019 in a travel-associated transmission cluster. MedRXiv. March 8, 2020. https://doi.org/10.1101/2020.03.05.20030502
2. Asadi S, Bouvier N, Wexler AS, Ristenpart WD. The coronavirus pandemic and aerosols: Does COVID-19 transmit via expiratory particles?Aerosol Science and Technology. 2020. https://www.tandfonline.com/doi/full/10.1080/02786826.2020.1749229
3. Wölfel R, Corman VM, Guggemos W, et al. Virological assessment of hospitalized cases of coronavirus disease 2019. MedRXiv. March 8, 2020. https://www.medrxiv.org/content/10.1101/2020.03.05.20030502v1.full.pdf
4. Worldometers.info, https://www.worldometers.info/coronavirus/coron avirus-age-sex-demographics/ Accessed April 8, 2020
5. Personal communication.
6. Fang L, Karakiulakis G, Roth M. Are patients with hypertension and diabetes mellitus at increased risk for COVID-19 infection? Lancet. Published online March 11, 2020. https://www.thelancet.com/action/showPdf?pii=S2213-2600%2820%2930116-8
7. Zhang R, Wang X, Ni L, et al. COVID-19: Melatonin as a potential adjuvant treatment. Life Sciences. 1 June 2020;250:117583. https://www.sciencedirect.com/science/article/pii/S0024320520303313
8. Ignatowska-Jankowska B, Jankowski M, Glac W, Swiergel AH. Cannabidiol-induced lymphopenia does not involve NKT and NK cells. J Physiol Pharmacol. 2009 Oct;60 Suppl 3:99-103. https://www.ncbi.nlm.nih.gov/pubmed/19996489
9. Trends in Pneumonia and Influenza Morbidity and Mortality American Lung Association Epidemiology and Statistics Unit Research and Health Education Division November 2015. https://www.lung.org/getmedia/98f088b5-3fd7-4c43-a490-ba8f4747bd4d/pi-trend-report.pdf.pdf Accessed April 8, 2020.
10. Centers for Disease Control. https://www.cdc.gov/nchs/nvss/vsrr/COVID19/ Accessed April 8, 2020.
11. Report of the WHO China Joint Mission on Coronavirus Disease 2019 (COVID-19). February 2020. https://www.who.int/docs/default-source/coronaviruse/who-china-joint-mission-on-covid-19-final-report.pdf Accessed on April 8, 2020.
12. Gorbalenya AE. Severe acute respiratory syndrome-related coronavirus (The species and its viruses, a statement of the Coronavirus Study Group. February 11, 2020. https://doi.org/10.1101/2020.02.07.937862. Accessed: February 13, 2020.
13. Centers for Disease Control. Situation Summary. February 29, 2020. https://www.cdc.gov/coronavirus/2019-ncov/summary.html. Accessed April 8, 2020.
14. Wei WE, Li Z, Chiew CJ, Yong SE, Toh MP, Lee VJ. Presymptomatic Transmission of SARS-CoV-2 — Singapore, January 23–March 16, 2020. MMWR Morb Mortal Wkly Rep. April 1, 2020. https://www.cdc.gov/mmwr/volumes/69/wr/mm6914e1.htm
15. Xiao F, Tang M, Zheng X, et al. Evidence for gastrointestinal infection of SARS-COV-2. Gastroenterology. 2020. doi: https://doi.org/10.1053/j.gastro.2020.02.055

16. Yeo C, Kaushal S, Yeo D. Enteric involvement of coronaviruses: is faecal-oral transmission of SARS-CoV-2 possible? Lancet Gastroenterol Hepatol. 2020 Apr;5(4):335-7.
https://www.thelancet.com/journals/langas/article/PII S2468-1253(20)30048-0/fulltext

17. Brann DH, Tsukahara T, Weinreb C, et al. Non-neural expression of SARS-CoV-2 entry genes in the olfactory epithelium suggests mechanisms underlying anosmia in COVID-19 patients. bioRxiv. March 28, 2020.
https://www.biorxiv.org/content/10.1101/2020.03.25.0 09084v2

18. Wan Y, Shang J, Graham R, Baric RS, Li F. Receptor recognition by novel coronavirus from Wuhan: An analysis based on decade-long structural studies of SARS. J Virology 2020; published online Jan 29.
https://www.ncbi.nlm.nih.gov/pubmed/31996437

19. Li XC, Zhang J, Zhuo JL. The vasoprotective axes of the renin-angiotensin system: physiological relevance and therapeutic implications in cardiovascular, hypertensive and kidney diseases. Pharmacol Res. 2017 Nov;125(Pt A):21-38. doi: 10.1016/j.phrs.2017.06.005.

20. Ding H-G, Deng Y-Y, Yang R-q. Hypercapnia induces IL-1β overproduction via activation of NLRP3 inflammasome: implication in cognitive impairment in hypoxemic adult rats. J Neuroinflammation. 2018.15(4).
https://link.springer.com/article/10.1186/s12974-017-1051-y

21. Li D, Ren W, Jiang Z, Zhu L. Regulation of the NLRP3 inflammasome and macrophage pyroptosis by the p38 MAPK signaling pathway in a mouse model of acute lung injury. Mol Med Rep. 2018 Nov; 18(5): 4399-4409.
https://www.ncbi.nlm.nih.gov/pmc/articles/PMC6172370/

22. Grailer JJ, Canning BA, Kalbitz M, et al. Critical role for the NLRP3 inflammasome during acute lung injury. J Immunol. 2014 Jun 15;192(12):5974-83.
https://www.ncbi.nlm.nih.gov/pmc/articles/PMC4061751/

23. Hui DS, I Azhar E, Madani TA, et al. The continuing 2019-nCoV epidemic threat of novel coronaviruses to global health - The latest 2019 novel coronavirus outbreak in Wuhan, China. Int J Infect Dis. 2020 Jan 14;91:264-6.
https://www.ncbi.nlm.nih.gov/pubmed/31953166

24. Huang C, Wang Y, Li X, et al. Clinical features of patients infected with 2019 novel coronavirus in Wuhan, China. Lancet. 2020 Feb 15;395(10223):497-506.
https://www.ncbi.nlm.nih.gov/pubmed/31986264

25. Bogoch II, Watts A, Thomas-Bachli A, et al. Pneumonia of Unknown Etiology in Wuhan, China: Potential for International Spread Via Commercial Air Travel. J Travel Med. 2020 Mar 13;27(2). pii: taaa008.
https://www.ncbi.nlm.nih.gov/pubmed/31943059

26. Huang C, Wang Y, Li X, et al. Clinical features of patients infected with 2019 novel coronavirus in Wuhan, China. Lancet. 2020 Feb 15;395(10223):497-506.
https://www.ncbi.nlm.nih.gov/pubmed/31986264

27. Wei M, Yuan J, Liu Y, et al. Novel Coronavirus Infection in Hospitalized Infants Under 1 Year of Age in China. JAMA. 2020 Feb 14. [Epub Ahead of Print]. doi: 10.1001/jama.2020.2131.

28. Zou L, Ruan F, Huang M, et al. SARS-CoV-2 Viral Load in Upper Respiratory Specimens of Infected Patients. N Engl J Med. 2020 Mar 19;382(12):1177-9.
https://www.ncbi.nlm.nih.gov/pubmed/32074444

29. Li Q, Guan X, Wu P, et al. Early Transmission Dynamics in Wuhan, China, of Novel Coronavirus-Infected Pneumonia. N Engl J Med. 2020 Mar 26;382(13):1199-1207. https://www.ncbi.nlm.nih.gov/pubmed/31995857

30. CDC Health Alert Network. Update and Interim Guidance on Outbreak of 2019 Novel Coronavirus (2019-nCoV) in Wuhan, China. CDC. January 17, 2020 https://emergency.cdc.gov/han/han00426.asp. Accessed: January 27, 2020.

31. Coronavirus Disease 2019 (COVID-19): COVID-19 Situation Summary. CDC. February 29, 2020 https://www.cdc.gov/coronavirus/2019-ncov/summary.html. Accessed: March 2, 2020

32. Shen C, Wang Z, Zhao F, et al. Treatment of 5 Critically Ill Patients With COVID-19 With Convalescent Plasma. JAMA. Published online March 27, 2020. doi:10.1001/jama.2020.4783

33. Zimmer C. Scientists Identify 69 Drugs to Test Against the Coronavirus. New York Times. https://www.nytimes.com/2020/03/22/science/coronavirus-drugs-chloroquine.html Accessed April 8, 2020.

34. Gautret P, Lagier JC, Parola P, et al. Hydroxychloroquine and azithromycin as a treatment of COVID-19: results of an open-label non-randomized clinical trial. Int J Antimicrob Agents. 2020 Mar 20:105949. [Epub Ahead of Print.] https://www.sciencedirect.com/science/article/pii/S0924857920300996

35. Huixia S, Yin D. Reporters notebook: life and death in a Wuhan coronavirus ICU. The Straits Times. https://www.straitstimes.com/asia/east-asia/reporters-notebook-life-and-death-in-a-wuhan-coronavirus-icu Accessed April 9, 2020.

36. Huijskens MJ, Walczak M, Koller N, et al. Technical advance: ascorbic acid induces development of double-positive T cells from human hematopoietic stem cells in the absence of stromal cells. J Leukoc Biol. 2014 Dec;96(6):1165-75.

37. Manning J, Mitchell B, Appadurai DA, et al. Vitamin C Promotes Maturation of T-Cells. Antioxid Redox Signal. 2013 Dec 10;19(17):2054-67. https://www.ncbi.nlm.nih.gov/pmc/articles/PMC3869442

38. Huijskens MJ, Walczak M, Sarkar S, et al. Ascorbic acid promotes proliferation of natural killer cell populations in culture systems applicable for natural killer cell therapy. Cytotherapy. 2015 May;17(5):613-20. https://www.ncbi.nlm.nih.gov/pubmed/25747742/

39. Article in Chinese. https://mp.weixin.qq.com/s/bF2YhJKiOfe1yimBc4XwOA Accessed April 8, 2020.

40. Article in Chinese. http://2yuan.xjtu.edu.cn/Html/News/Articles/21774.html. Accessed April 8, 2020.

41. Gonzalez MJ, Berdiel MJ, Duconge J, et al. High dose vitamin C and influenza: A case report. J Orthomol Med. 2018 Jun;33(3). https://isom.ca/article/high-dose-vitamin-c-influenza-case-report.

42. Gorton HC, Jarvis K. The effectiveness of vitamin C in preventing and relieving the symptoms of virus-induced respiratory infections. J Manip Physiol Ther. 1999;22:8, 530-3. https://www.ncbi.nlm.nih.gov/pubmed/10543583

43. Hemilä H. Vitamin C and infections. Nutrients. 2017;9(4). pii:E339. https://www.ncbi.nlm.nih.gov/pubmed/28353648

44. Hickey S, Saul AW. Vitamin C: The real story. Basic Health Pub. October 23, 2015. ISBN-13: 978-1591202233.

45. Kim Y, Kim H, Bae S, et al. Vitamin C is an essential factor on the anti-viral immune responses through the production of interferon-α/β at the initial stage of influenza A virus (H3N2) infection. Immune Netw. 2013;13:70-74. https://www.ncbi.nlm.nih.gov/pubmed/23700397

46. Hunt C, Chakravorty NK, Annan G, et al. The clinical effects of vitamin C supplementation in elderly hospitalised patients with acute respiratory infections. Int J Vitam Nutr Res. 1994;64:212-9.
47. Ren Shiguang, et al. Hebei Medicine. 1978,4:1-3.
48. Hemilä H, Chalker E. Vitamin C can shorten the length of stay in the ICU: A meta-analysis. Nutrients. 2019 Mar 27;11:4. pii: E708. doi: 10.3390/nu11040708.
49. Hemilä H, Chalker E. Vitamin C Can Shorten the Length of Stay in the ICU: A Meta-Analysis. Nutrients. 2019 Mar 27;11(4). pii: E708. https://www.ncbi.nlm.nih.gov/pubmed/30934660 e
50. Khan IM, et al. Efficacy of vitamin C in reducing duration of severe pneumonia in children. J Rawalpindi Med Coll (JRMC). 2014;18(1):55-7. https://www.journalrmc.com/index.php/JRMC/article/view/381/290
51. Stone I. Hypoascorbemia: The genetic disease causing the human requirement for exogenous ascorbic acid. Perspect Biol Med. 1966;10:133-4. https://www.ncbi.nlm.nih.gov/pubmed/6002772
52. Subramanian, N. et al. Detoxification of histamine with ascorbic acid. Biochem Pharmacol. 1973;27:1671-3.
53. National Institutes of Health. Vitamin C. Fact Sheet for Professionals. https://ods.od.nih.gov/factsheets/VitaminC-HealthProfessional/ Accessed April 9, 2020.
54. Cathcart RF. Vitamin C Can Shorten the Length of Stay in the ICU: A Meta-Analysis. Medical Hypotheses. 1981;7(11):1359-76. https://www.ncbi.nlm.nih.gov/pubmed/7321921
55. Farrell SE. Acetaminophen Toxicity. January 17, 2020. Medscape. http://www.emedicine.com/ped/topic7.htm Accessed April 9, 2020.
56. Oregon State University. https://lpi.oregonstate.edu/sites/lpi.oregonstate.edu/files/pdf/lpi_vitamin_c_special_statement_on_covid-19.pdf Accessed April 9, 2020.
57. Registered clinical trials on Vitamin C and COVID-19. https://clinicaltrials.gov/ct2/show/NCT04264533 Accessed April 9, 2020.
58. Chronobiology. Studies Show Melatonin May Help Fight Coronavirus. https://www.chronobiology.com/studies-show-melatonin-may-help-fight-coronavirus/ Accessed April 9, 2020.
59. Grivas TB, Savvidou OD. Melatonin the "light of night" in human biology and adolescent idiopathic scoliosis. Scoliosis. 2007;2:6. https://www.ncbi.nlm.nih.gov/pubmed/?term=%22Savvidou+AND+Melatonin+AND+200 7%22
60. Rahim I, Djerdjouri B, Sayed RK, et al. Melatonin administration to wild-type mice and nontreated NLRP3 mutant mice share similar inhibition of the inflammatory response during sepsis. J Pineal Res. First published: 31 March 2017. https://doi.org/10.1111/jpi.12410
61. Rodríguez MI, Escames G, López LC, et al. Chronic melatonin treatment reduces the age-dependent inflammatory process in senescence-accelerated mice. J Pineal Res. 2007;42(3):272-9. https://doi.org/10.1111/j.1600-079X.2006.00416.x
62. Kumar V. Inflammasomes: Pandora's box for sepsis. J Inflamm Res. 2018 Dec 11;11:477-502. doi: 10.2147/JIR.S178084.
63. Acuña-Castroviejo D, Carretero M, Doerrier C, et al. Melatonin protects lung mitochondria from aging. AGE. 2012; 34:681-92. https://doi.org/10.1007/s11357-011-9267-8
64. Wu G, Peng C, Liao W, et al. Melatonin receptor agonist protects against acute lung injury induced by ventilator through up-regulation of IL-10 production. Respir Res. 2020;21:65. https://doi.org/10.1186/s12931-020-1325-2

65. Zhang R, Wang X, Ni L, et al. COVID-19: Melatonin as a potential adjuvant treatment. Life Sci. 2020 June; 250; 117583. https://www.sciencedirect.com/science/article/pii/S0024320520303313

66. Sun CK, Lee FY,, Kao YH, et al. Systemic combined melatonin-mitochondria treatment improves acute respiratory distress syndrome in the rat J. Pineal Res. 2015; 58:137-50. 10.1111/jpi.12199

67. Ling Y, Li ZZ, Zhang JF, et al. MicroRNA-494 inhibition alleviates acute lung injury through Nrf2 signaling pathway via NQO1 in sepsis-associated acute respiratory distress syndrome. Life Sci. 2018;210:1-8. 10.1016/j.lfs.2018.08.037

68. Pedrosa AM, Weinlich R, Mognol GP, et al. Melatonin protects CD4+ T cells from activation-induced cell death by blocking NFAT-mediated CD95 ligand upregulation J. Immunol. 2010;184:3487-94. doi: 10.4049/jimmunol.0902961

69. Shang Y, Xu SP, Wu Y, et al. Melatonin reduces acute lung injury in endotoxemic rats. Chin Med J (Engl). 2009;122(12):1388-93. https://www.ncbi.nlm.nih.gov/pubmed/?term=%22Melatonin+reduces+acute+lung+injury+in+endotoxemic+rats%22

70. Ahmadi Z, Ashrafizadeh M. Melatonin as a potential modulator of Nrf2. Fundam Clin Pharmacol. 2020;34(1):11-19. doi: 10.1111/fcp.12498

71. Habtemariam S, Daglia M, Sureda A, et al. Melatonin and respiratory diseases: a review. Curr Top Med Chem. 2017;17:467-88. http://www.eurekaselect.com/145042/article

72. Sundaram ME, Coleman LA. Vitamin D and Influenza. Adv Nutr. 2012 Jul;3(4):517-25. doi: 10.3945/an.112.002162.

73. Cannell JJ, Vieth R, Umhau JC, et al. Epidemic influenza and vitamin D. Epidemiol Infect. 2006;134:1129-40. https://www.ncbi.nlm.nih.gov/pubmed/16959053

74. RCannell JJ, Zasloff M, Garland CF, et al. On the epidemiology of influenza. Virol J. 2008;5:29. https://www.ncbi.nlm.nih.gov/pubmed/16959053.

75. Ginde AA, Mansbach JM, Camargo CA Jr. Association between serum 25-hydroxyvitamin D level and upper respiratory tract infection in the Third National Health and Nutrition Examination Survey. Arch Intern Med. 2009;169:384-90. https://www.ncbi.nlm.nih.gov/pubmed/19237723.

76. Martineau AR, Jolliffe DA, Hooper RL, et al. Vitamin D supplementation to prevent acute respiratory tract infections: systematic review and meta-analysis of individual participant data. BMJ. 2017;356:i6583. https://www.ncbi.nlm.nih.gov/pubmed/28202713.

77. Martineau AR. Vitamin D supplementation to prevent acute respiratory tract infections: systematic review and meta-analysis of individual participant data. BMJ. 2017 Feb 15;356:i6583. doi: 10.1136/bmj.i6583.

78. Urashima M, Segawa T, Okazaki M, et al. Randomized trial of vitamin D supplementation to prevent seasonal influenza A in schoolchildren. Am J Clin Nutr. 2010;91:1255-60. https://www.ncbi.nlm.nih.gov/pubmed/20219962.

79. Arihiro S, Nakashima A, Matsuoka M, et al. Randomized Trial of Vitamin D Supplementation to Prevent Seasonal Influenza and Upper Respiratory Infection in Patients With Inflammatory Bowel Disease. Inflamm Bowel Dis. 2019 Jun;25(6):1088-95. .gov/pmc/articles/PMC6499936/

80. Loeb M, Dang AD, Thiem VD, et al. Effect of Vitamin D supplementation to reduce respiratory infections in children and adolescents in Vietnam: A randomized controlled trial. Influenza Other Respir Viruses. 2019 Mar;13(2):176-83. https://www.ncbi.nlm.nih.gov/pmc/articles/PMC6379634/

81. Zhou J, Du J, Huang L, et al. Preventive Effects of Vitamin D on Seasonal Influenza A in Infants: A Multicenter, Randomized, Open, Controlled Clinical Trial. Pediatr Infect Dis J. 2018;37(8):749-54. https://www.ncbi.nlm.nih.gov/pmc/articles/PMC4463890/
82. Long S, Romani AM. Role of cellular magnesium in human diseases. Austin J Nutr Food Sci. 2014;2(10):1051. http://austinpublishinggroup.com/nutrition-food-sciences/fulltext/ajnfs-v2-id1051.php
83. McCarthy JT, Kumar R. "Divalent cation metabolism: magnesium," in Schrier R (series ed.), The Atlas of Diseases of the Kidney, Blackwell, Oxfordshire, 1999.
84. Heaton FW. "Role of magnesium in enzyme systems," in Siegel H (ed.), Metal Ions in Biologic Systems, Marcel Dekker, New York, 1990.]
85. de Baaij JHF, JGJ Hoenderop, RJM Bindels. Magnesium in man: Implications for health and disease. Physiol Rev. 2015 Jan;95(1):1-46. http://physrev.physiology.org/content/95/1/1.long
86. Rosanoff A. The Essential Nutrient Magnesium -Key to Mitochondrial ATP Production and Much More. ProHealth. June 8, 2009. https://www.prohealth.com/library/print.cfm?libid=14606 Accessed April 9, 2020.
87. Abraham GE, Flechas JD. Management of fibromyalgia: rationale for the use of magnesium and malic acid. J Nutr Med. 1992;3:49-59. https://www.ncbi.nlm.nih.gov/pubmed/8587088
88. Fraker PJ, King LE, Laakko T, Vollmer TL. The dynamic link between the integrity of the immune system and zinc status. J Nutr. 2000;130:1399S-406S. https://www.ncbi.nlm.nih.gov/pubmed/10801951
89. Liu MJ, Bao S, Gálvez-Peralta M, et al. ZIP8 regulates host defense through zinc-mediated inhibition of NF-κB. Cell Rep. 2013;3:386-400. https://www.ncbi.nlm.nih.gov/pubmed/23403290
90. Shankar AH, Prasad AS. Zinc and immune function: the biological basis of altered resistance to infection. Am J Clin Nutr. 1998;68:447S-463S. https://www.ncbi.nlm.nih.gov/pubmed/9701160
91. Hoffmann PR, Berry MJ. The influence of selenium on immune responses. Mol Nutr Food Res. 2008;52:1273-80. https://www.ncbi.nlm.nih.gov/pubmed/18384097
92. Steinbrenner H, Al-Quraishy S, Dkhil MA, et al. Dietary selenium in adjuvant therapy of viral and bacterial infections. Adv Nutr. 2015;6:73-82. https://www.ncbi.nlm.nih.gov/pubmed/25593145
93. Food and Drug Administration. FDA Approves First Drug Comprised of an Active Ingredient Derived from Marijuana to Treat Rare, Severe Forms of Epilepsy.https://www.fda.gov/news-events/press-announcements/fda-approves-first-drug-comprised-active-ingredient-derived-marijuana-treat-rare-severe-forms. Accessed April 9, 2020.
94. Lachenmeier DW, Habel S, Fischer B, et al. Are side effects of cannabidiol (CBD) products caused by tetrahydrocannabinol (THC) contamination?F1000Res. 2019 Aug 8;8:1394. doi: 10.12688/f1000research.19931.2
95. Irving PM, Iqbal T, Nwokolo C, et al. A Randomized, Double-blind, Placebo-controlled, Parallel-group, Pilot Study of Cannabidiol-rich Botanical Extract in the Symptomatic Treatment of Ulcerative Colitis. Inflamm Bowel Dis. 2018 Mar 19;24(4):714-24. doi: 10.1093/ibd/izy002
96. Wu HJ, Wu E. The role of gut microbiota in immune homeostasis and autoimmunity. Gut Microbes. 2012 Jan 1;3(1):4-14. doi: 10.4161/gmic.19320
97. Cani PD, Plovier H, Van Hul M, et al. Endocannabinoids--at the crossroads between the gut microbiota and host metabolism. Nat Rev Endocrinol. 2016 Mar;12(3):133-43. doi: 10.1038/nrendo.2015.211

98. Yao X, Ye F, Zhang M, et al. In Vitro Antiviral Activity and Projection of Optimized Dosing Design of Hydroxychloroquine for the Treatment of Severe Acute Respiratory Syndrome Coronavirus 2 (SARS-CoV-2). Clinical Infectious Diseases. 2020 Mar 9.
https://doi.org/10.1093/cid/ciaa237

99. Rossignol JF. Nitazoxanide, a new drug candidate for the treatment of Middle East respiratory syndrome coronavirus. J Infect Public Health. 2016;9(3):227-30.
https://doi.org/10.1016/j.jiph.2016.04.001.

100. Yao T-T, Qian J-D, Zhu W-Y, et al. A systematic review of lopinavir therapy for SARS coronavirus and MERS coronavirus—A possible reference for coronavirus disease-19 treatment option. J Med Virol. 2020;1- 8.
https://doi.org/10.1002/jmv.25729

101. Blázquez-Prieto J, Huidobro C, López-Alonso I, et al. Cellular senescence limits acute lung injury induced by mechanical ventilation. bioRXiv. 2020 Mar 25.
https://www.biorxiv.org/content/10.1101/2020.03.24.0 05983v1

102. Moskowitz JM. We have no reason to believe 5G is safe. Scientific American. October 17, 2019.
https://blogs.scientificamerican.com/observations/we-have-no-reason-to-believe-5g-is-safe/ Accessed April 9, 2020.

103. Donahue JG, Kieke BA, King JP, et al. Association of spontaneous abortion with receipt of inactivated influenza vaccine containing H1N1pdm09 in 2010-11 and 2011-12. Vaccine. 2017 Sep 25;35(40):5314-22.
https://www.ncbi.nlm.nih.gov/pubmed/28917295

104. Miller E, Andrews N, Stellitano L, et al. Risk of narcolepsy in children and young people receiving AS03 adjuvanted pandemic A/H1N1 2009 influenza vaccine: retrospective analysis. BMJ. 2013 Feb 26;346:f794.
https://www.ncbi.nlm.nih.gov/pubmed/23444425/

105. Sarkanen T, Alakuijala A, Julkunen I, Partinen M. Narcolepsy Associated with Pandemrix Vaccine. Curr Neurol Neurosci Rep. 2018 Jun 1;18(7):43.
https://www.ncbi.nlm.nih.gov/pubmed/29855798

106. Dauvilliers Y, Arnulf I, Lecendreux M, et al. Increased risk of narcolepsy in children and adults after pandemic H1N1 vaccination in France. Brain. 2013 Aug;136(Pt 8):2486-96.
https://www.ncbi.nlm.nih.gov/pubmed/23884811

107. O'Flanagan D, Barret AS, Foley M, et al. Investigation of an association between onset of narcolepsy and vaccination with pandemic influenza vaccine, Ireland April 2009-December 2010. Euro Surveill. 2014 May 1;19(17):15-25.
https://www.ncbi.nlm.nih.gov/pubmed/24821121

108. Trogstad L, Bakken IJ, Gunnes N, et al. Narcolepsy and hypersomnia in Norwegian children and young adults following the influenza A(H1N1) 2009 pandemic. Vaccine. 2017 Apr 4;35(15):1879-85.
https://www.ncbi.nlm.nih.gov/pubmed/28302408

109. Mahajan D, Cook J, McIntyre PB, et al. Annual report: surveillance of adverse events following immunisation in Australia, 2010. Commun Dis Intell Q Rep. 2011 Dec;35(4):263-80.
https://www.ncbi.nlm.nih.gov/pubmed/22624487

110. Idrus AA. Biopharma's no-holds-barred fight to find a COVID-19 vaccine: The full list. March 20, 2020.
https://www.fiercebiotech.com/biotech/biopharma-s-no-holds-barred-fight-to-find-a-covid-19-vaccine-full-list

111. Public Health Emergency. Public Readiness and Emergency Preparedness Act.
https://www.phe.gov/Preparedness/legal/prepact/Pages/default.aspx Accessed April 9, 2020.

112. FDA. Fact Sheet: FDA at a Glance.
https://www.fda.gov/about-fda/fda-basics/fact-sheet-fda-glance Accessed April 9, 2020.

113. World Health Organization. Seventy-First World Health Assembly. Voluntary contributions by fund and by contributor, 2017. http://apps.who.int/gb/ebwha/pdf_files/WHA71/A71_INF2Corr1-en.pdf Accessed April 9, 2020.

114. Taylor G. GreenMedInfo. Examining RFK Jr's claim that the CDC "owns over 20 vaccine patents." January 17, 2017. https://www.greenmedinfo.com/blog/examining-rfk-jrs-claim-cdc-owns-over-20-vaccine-patents Accessed April 9, 2020.

115. HHS.gov. HHS fiscal year 2018 budget in brief -CDC. https://www.hhs.gov/about/budget/fy2018/budget-in-brief/cdc/index.html Accessed April 9, 2020.

116. Bao L, Deng W, Gao H, et al. Reinfection could not occur in SARS-CoV-2 infected rhesus macaques. bioRXiv. 2020 Mar 14. https://www.biorxiv.org/content/10.1101/2020.03.13.99 0226v1

117. Oregon Health & Science University. https://news.ohsu.edu/2020/04/04/preparing-for-the-novel-coronavirus-at-ohsu. Accessed April 9, 2020.

118. Wolff GG. Influenza vaccination and respiratory virus interference among Department of Defense personnel during the 2017–2018 influenza season. Vaccine. 2020;38;350-4.

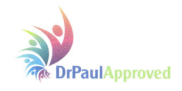

APPENDIX A
OTHER IMPORTANT RESOURCES

Get the latest public health information from CDC: https://www.coronavirus.gov .

Get the latest research from NIH: https://www.nih.gov/coronavirus.

WHO Coronavirus resources: https://www.who.int/health-topics/coronavirus

WorldHealthOrganization Coronavirus Situation Dashboard: https://experience.arcgis.com/experience/685d0ace521648f8a5beeeee1b9125cd

CDC COVID-19 page: https://www.cdc.gov/coronavirus/2019-ncov/cases-updates/testing-in-us.html?CDC_AA_refVal=https%3A%2F%2Fwww.cdc.gov%2Fcoronavirus%2F2019-ncov%2Ftesting-in-us.html

Johns Hopkins Coronavirus Resource Center: https://coronavirus.jhu.edu

Prediction models for deaths in the USA - when it will peak: https://covid19.healthdata.org/projections

World Link Journal Club Presentation with two key papers: https://www.worldlinkmedical.com/covid-19-update-neal-rouzier/

American Lung Association Paper: The real influenza and pneumonia rates – "Trends in Pneumonia and Influenza Morbidity and Mortality" https://www.lung.org/getmedia/98f088b5-3fd7-4c43-a490-ba8f4747bd4d/pi-trend-report.pdf.pdf

The information in this book is educational and Informational only: IT IS NOT MEDICAL ADVICE. It is not intended to diagnose or treat. No pharmaceutical or dietary supplement has been proven in long-term placebo-controlled studies to treat or prevent COVID-19.